Stephen C Smith DDS

KILLING PAIN
WITHOUT
PRESCRIPTION

KILLING PAIN WITHOUT PRESCRIPTION

A New and Simple Way to Free
Yourself from Headache, Backache,
and Other Sources of Chronic Pain

HAROLD GELB, D.M.D.
PAULA M. SIEGEL

HARPER & ROW, PUBLISHERS

NEW YORK

Cambridge
Hagerstown
Philadelphia
San Francisco

1817

London
Mexico City
São Paulo
Sydney

FIRST EDITION

Designer: Janice Stern

Library of Congress Cataloging in Publication Data

Gelb, Harold.
  Killing pain without prescription.

  Includes index.
    1. Pain—Prevention.   2. Muscle rigidity.
3. Relaxation.   I. Siegel, Paula M., joint author.
II. Title.
RB128.G44   616'.047   79–2619
ISBN 0–06–011483–5

80 81 82 83 10 9 8 7 6 5 4 3 2 1

To all the unfortunate chronic pain patients, many of whom can now look forward to a life free of suffering

Contents

Preface

The most difficult part of my practice is listening to the desperate plaints of my patients. Even after hearing the same stories for thirty years, I am still filled with consternation when I listen to what these people, with essentially simple problems, have suffered. The physiology of their pain should not be difficult for a medical professional to understand. However, at present it falls outside the recognized medical protocol to diagnose a single pain by examining the whole body. You must develop new treatment guidelines. You must spend more time listening to the patient. And you need to rely on other health specialists as well. Voices in the medical community rise in indignation when the authority of the individual practitioner is threatened. Yet in multidisciplinary medicine, if patients are allowed to tell their story, they usually not only tell you what is wrong but how to be treated.

In this book, you have a blueprint for a new approach to pain. Our list of specialists may not be helpful to readers not living in major cities. They may find that physicians and dentists alike tend to be rigid in their treatment philosophies. A patient questioning their methods may not be welcomed with open arms. However, what is true in big business is true in the doctor/patient relationship. If the consumer is vocal about the need for a service, the supplier will eventually meet that need in order to keep the consumer's confidence.

I hope that this book will help you find a lasting relief from whatever discomfort you suffer. And in the end, perhaps it will give impetus to a medical movement that will prevent pain rather than treat it.

Acknowledgments

A book of this scope must attempt to overcome some of the shortcomings of our traditional, specialized health care system by crossing specialty and professional boundaries. Scientific isolationism undermines the development of a holistic approach to diagnosis and treatment of pain and dysfunction, the need for which is such a pressing problem for many individuals. Consequently, we found it necessary to confer with health professionals in many diverse fields to present a multi-disciplinary approach to this multi-factored disorder.

Those health professionals who directly or indirectly contributed greatly to the contents herein are: Hans Kraus, M.D., Janet Travell, M.D., Lila Wallis, M.D., Yale Palchick, D.D.S., Lawrence Funt, D.D.S., Brendan Stack, D.D.S., Sheldon Sinett, D.C., George Eversaul, Ph.D., Paul Mandl, Samuel Bursuk, Edna Lay, D.O., George Goodheart, D.C., Mariano Rocabado, P.T.

Introduction

This is a book of hope. For those of you with headaches, backaches, neckaches, shoulder aches—aches of a muscular nature anywhere in the body—the information in these pages can help you find relief. We're not talking about drugs that will mask symptoms, or mental exercises to help you live with the pain. This book will tell you how to treat the source of pain—the sore, tense muscles themselves.

The wealth of knowledge in this book does not come from my experience alone. I have gone to pain specialists in every field of medicine and, with their cooperation, developed an approach to pain using all our ideas. I've talked with neurologists, psychiatrists, orthopedists, physical therapists, osteopaths, nutritionists, biofeedback clinicians and many more medical professionals, all of whom have different answers to the pain problem. We found that working together on every patient brought our success rate up to 85 or 90 percent in relieving pain where we had failed before. The key was in treating the patient as a whole unit in which all the parts are interrelated and interdependent.

I am going to share our knowledge with you in this book. We'll discuss the origin of muscular pain—the kind of pain that is responsible for 90 percent of our aches. A nutritionist will tell you why your diet aggravates a pain problem and how you can change your eating habits to diminish discomfort. Biofeedback will be explained, along with some exercises you can use at home. We'll talk about physical exercise and what kind of workout is best for you as well as which activities you should shy away from.

As you can see, the program I use for relieving pain depends a great deal on my patients' willingness to take control of their problem. In this book, I'm not only going to tell you where to get professional help for your pain; I'm going to give you the fundamentals for altering your habits to start the healing now. Up to over *half* of the pain source could be in what you eat, how you sit, how much exercise—any number of factors that *you* can change.

You can play so important a role in relieving your pain because the kind of pain most of us suffer is due to muscle-contraction or muscle-tension disorder. Unlike discomfort due to disease or some biochemical imbalance, muscle-tension pain can be controlled. You can learn to relax the muscles and to cope with stress more effectively so that you don't tense up under strain. You can exercise to keep the muscles healthy. Once recognized, this kind of chronic pain is actually the easiest to relieve with proper care.

Proper care begins with a new approach to the problem. When you have a chronic headache, you'll no longer think of it as just a pain in the head. You'll regard that discomfort, as well as any other constant pain, as a distress signal from the whole body. The signal means that an imbalance exists in your body. It could be a hormonal imbalance, for instance, if you're taking a contraceptive pill. It could be a structural imbalance if one of your legs is slightly shorter than the other or if your jaws are unbalanced. You might even find that the way you hold your body causes the pain. If you're always cupping the phone between shoulder and chin while taking notes or working with your hands, your shoulder, neck and head muscles could be tight. Physical imbalances and poor posture habits cause the muscles to tense up and stay that way. If you add emotional stress to these physical strains, the muscles will tighten up to the point where they become painful.

In our approach to pain, you wouldn't take a pill or other harmful medication to relax the muscles or dull the ache. You'd remove the stressful stimulus—discontinue taking the Pill, balance out the leg lengths, reposition the jaw, or learn to hold the phone with one hand

and keep the other hand free for note-taking or other activity. You take away the tension-causing factor; you don't compensate for it with drugs. In other words, we believe that you should work with the body, not against it, to relieve pain. Pain means that something is amiss in the body. If you correct the imbalance, the discomfort will disappear. However, if you simply mask *over* the ache with drugs and continue to abuse the body, the pain will continue and intensify.

Sounds like a logical approach to this problem, doesn't it? But how many times have you developed a headache during a stressful day and, rather than take five minutes out to relax, as your body was requesting, gulped down three or four aspirin tablets to keep going? How many times have you been commended for coming in to work or school, or attending a social function, despite a physical discomfort? We spend $25 billion a year in the search for relief of pain so that we can keep the shoulder to the grindstone. Most of these dollars go toward drugs and operations to hide or cut the pain. Since they don't usually remove the cause of the discomfort, these procedures work temporarily if at all. So every few months we shop for a new doctor and treatment, some of which are innocuous and some harmful. None, however, give lasting relief.

To help the pain sufferer off this medical treadmill, we've sought out and discovered a more promising treatment for pain by working with the whole person, body and mind. Most exemplary of this new approach are the pain clinics formed and forming around the country. The clinics often devote themselves to weaning patients off painkillers, finding the source of the pain, and working with the body's own integrity to relieve the discomfort.

Take backache clinics, for example. Thousands of low-back-pain victims are operated upon unsuccessfully every year. When they're not in surgery, they're living on drugs. Yet neither of these treatments addresses the cause of the problem—tense muscles. Those patients who finally enter a back-pain clinic are given a battery of tests to find out where the muscles are strained and what is causing the tightness. In the majority of cases, the prescribed treatment includes: replacing drugs with ice packs or heat applications to relieve the pain; exercising to loosen, tone and rebuild knotted muscles; massaging to further help restore the tight muscles to their proper resilience; and learning some kind of stress-coping mechanism, like autohypnosis or biofeedback, to ward off future back problems.

In this country, we have three types of pain clinics: for headache, for backache and general chronic pain, and for temporomandibular joint dysfunction.

You're probably familiar with headache and backache, but what is the temporomandibular joint (TMJ)? This is the hinge that connects the upper and lower jaws. We have found that when the jaws become unbalanced, the resulting stress on the muscles in the body can cause head, neck, shoulder and back pain. Other problems, such as clogged ears and ringing or hissing noises, hormone imbalance and dizziness, have also been connected with this jaw imbalance, creating the TMJ Syndrome.

As you can see, many of the complaints precipitated by the TMJ imbalance are mistaken easily for other disorders. For instance, low-back pain and severe headaches that are part of the TMJ Syndrome often are misdiagnosed and improperly treated as spinal disk disorders or migraine headaches.

The confusion of the TMJ Syndrome with other pain problems would be reduced greatly if a test for this disorder were included in standard examinations for pain patients. Unfortunately, the medical world still considers the TMJ Syndrome to be a dental problem, affecting only the mouth. Uncovering the true nature of this disorder—that it affects the whole body—has taken many years of research. Only recently has the diagnosis of and treatment for the TMJ Syndrome filtered into the understanding of chronic pain.

Our findings about the manifestations of the TMJ Syndrome have provided us with a new key to controlling chronic pain. For millions of people, recognition of a TMJ imbalance can be the pivotal point in successful management of their pain. We estimate that one third of the American population has some medical problem exacerbated by a jaw imbalance. One third of the people in this country stand a chance of living healthier lives by recognizing the TMJ Syndrome, knowing how to relieve it, and taking preventive steps against it. In the following chapters, you'll find all the information you need to understand this common disorder. So without further delay . . .

KILLING PAIN
WITHOUT
PRESCRIPTION

1

Profile of a Chronic Pain Sufferer

Who suffers from chronic pain? Neurotic people? Angry people? Perfectionists? I'm sure that some of these kinds of people are victims of chronic pain, but certainly not all pain sufferers fall into these categories. Rich people and poor, intelligent and simple, emotional and calm, can all suffer persistent aches. Pain doesn't discriminate in choosing its victims.

Admittedly, some people do use their discomfort to get attention, seek revenge or avoid responsibility, but they make up only a small percentage of the chronic-pain population. Unfortunately, thousands of sufferers whose discomfort is physiological and offers them no emotional benefits are lumped together with the psychogenic-pain victims. Since the source of the discomfort is outside the working knowledge of a physician and/or specialist, this person is packed off to a psychiatrist to work through his or her need for a pain disorder.

Most of these ill-treated suffers have muscle-tension pain—neckache, headache or backache, for example. Chronic muscular discomfort is the most common and the most poorly understood disorder in the medical world today. As in the case of any other disease, there is a *psychological* component in its development, but we also know that physical, treatable causes exist apart from the emotional aspects.

Muscular disorders are usually induced by stress, whether that stress is caused by some body-structure imbalance or by an emotionally loaded event. The muscles will react in one or more of

1

four ways: (1) they will develop spasms; (2) they will lose their tone and become weak; (3) they will tense up; (4) trigger points will develop inside them (trigger points will be described in detail at the end of this chapter). When muscles develop any or all of these conditions, they become painful. And no amount of psychotherapy, drugs or surgery is going to relieve that pain permanently although it may help temporarily.

When I say that muscle tension causes most of the pain suffered in this country, I'm talking about seventy to eighty million individuals. How can so many people share the same disorder? Because the precipitating factor in most cases is stress. If there's one common psychological characteristic among these sufferers, it's their inability to cope with stress. Yet in our fast-paced, competitive society, who can escape pressure?

Internalizing Stress

Your ability to cope with stress is fairly well established at an early age. Even in four- or five-year-old children, you'll notice that some handle tense situations easily while others experience, say, stomach sickness, rashes or asthma attacks. A strong reactor to stress in childhood will probably carry that trait throughout life.

Many tension-related illnesses result from internalizing emotions. Instead of yelling back at the boss, you sit on the feelings. They have no way to be released unless they take over some bodily function.

Our physical response to stress, however, has not always been detrimental to our health. Human beings were cleverly designed to have a built-in reaction to outside stimuli. When there is a sudden noise or heightened emotional situation, the body will pump extra hormones into the system to speed up the heartbeat, increase blood pressure, tense the muscles and quicken breathing. Your whole body braces for action. In prehistoric times, you'd have been ready to pounce on the invader or leap out of danger's way.

Today we have countless more outside irritants than did primitive man—traffic, subways, stereos, office machinery, household appliances, TV. But none of these irritants is dangerous. Certainly, you're not supposed to go running into a corner when the vacuum cleaner is on. Nor are you supposed to run away from many potentially hazardous emotional situations—asking the boss for a raise, competing with someone for a position, inching along in rush-hour automobile traffic. Unfortunately, the body still prepares you to leave these situations in a flash and you constantly force yourself to go against those instincts. Since you're not releasing the tension that is building up in your body, it continues to accumulate until it's released as a headache, a backache or stomach cramps.

The relation of stress to illness has been researched extensively in the last decade. We've found that the more upheaval you have in your life, be it good or bad, the more prone to illness you'll be. In the table below,* you'll see one of the scales that have been developed to help researchers measure life stress and find out how much stress piles up before illness sets in. According to this scale, if you have a total of 200 stress points within a three-to-six-month period, the odds are about three to one that you'll become ill. If you score 300 or more, you have an 80 percent chance of developing a physical response to stress, which may even terminate in a nervous breakdown.

The Social Readjustment Rating Scale*

LIFE EVENT	MEAN VALUE	YOUR SCORE
1. Death of spouse	100	
2. Divorce	73	
3. Marital separation from mate	65	
4. Detention in jail or other institution	63	
5. Death of a close family member	63	
6. Major personal injury or illness	53	
7. Marriage	50	
8. Being fired at work	47	

*From Holmes, T. H. and Rahe, R. H.: The Social Readjustment Rating Scale. *Journal of Psychosomatic Research 11*: 213–218, 1967.

LIFE EVENT	MEAN VALUE	YOUR SCORE
9. Marital reconciliation with mate	45	
10. Retirement from work	45	
11. Major change in the health or behavior of a family member	44	
12. Pregnancy	40	
13. Sexual difficulties	39	
14. Gaining a new family member (e.g., through birth, adoption, oldster moving in, etc.)	39	
15. Major business readjustment (e.g., merger, reorganization, bankruptcy, etc.)	39	
16. Major change in financial state (e.g., a lot worse off or a lot better off than usual)	38	
17. Death of a close friend	37	
18. Changing to a different line of work	36	
19. Major change in the number of arguments with spouse (e.g., either a lot more or a lot less than usual regarding child-rearing, personal habits, etc.)	35	
20. Taking on a mortgage greater than $10,000 (e.g., purchasing a home, business, etc.)	31	
21. Foreclosure on a mortgage or loan	30	
22. Major change in responsibilities at work (e.g., promotion, demotion, lateral transfer)	29	
23. Son or daughter leaving home (e.g., marriage, attending college, etc.)	29	
24. In-law troubles	29	
25. Outstanding personal achievement	28	
26. Wife beginning or ceasing work outside the home	26	
27. Beginning or ceasing formal schooling	26	

LIFE EVENT	MEAN VALUE	YOUR SCORE
28. Major change in living conditions (e.g., building a new home, re-modeling, deterioration of home or neighborhood)	25	
29. Revision of personal habits (dress, manners, associations, etc.)	24	
30. Troubles with the boss	23	
31. Major change in working hours or conditions	20	
32. Change in residence	20	
33. Changing to a new school	20	
34. Major change in usual type and/or amount of recreation	19	
35. Major change in church activities (e.g., a lot more or a lot less than usual)	19	
36. Major change in social activities (e.g., clubs, dancing, movies, visiting, etc.)	18	
37. Taking on a mortgage or loan less than $10,000 (e.g., purchasing a car, TV, freezer, etc.)	17	
38. Major change in sleeping habits (a lot more or a lot less sleep, or change in part of day when asleep)	16	
39. Major change in number of family get-togethers (e.g., a lot more or a lot less than usual)	15	
40. Major change in eating habits (a lot more or a lot less food intake, or very different meal hours or surroundings)	15	
41. Vacation	13	
42. Christmas	12	
43. Minor violations of the law (e.g., traffic tickets, jaywalking, disturbing the peace, etc.)	11	

Stress can affect any part of the body, but it seems to have a preference for these five systems:

Gastrointestinal—If your emotions collect in this area, you'll probably suffer from chronic indigestion, nervous stomach, spastic colon, peptic ulcers or duodenal ulcers, to name a few of the common disorders.

Masticatory—As we all know, real men and brave women grit their teeth and go through with whatever unpleasant task is assigned to them. It's too bad that teeth weren't made to be gritted—or clenched or gnashed. Nonetheless, many people use their teeth to work off daily frustrations. If you're one of them, you've probably managed to force the jaws out of balance. Unbalanced jaws are a primary cause of chronic muscle pain in the head, neck and shoulders, as well as in the rest of the body. If you were to place this imbalance on the stress scale, it would be worth about 100 points. But unlike life events that cause stress for a certain, defined period of time, a jaw imbalance is not temporary. The strain it places on the body is a twenty-four-hour-a-day load, which can last a lifetime. Unbalanced jaws are a fairly recent discovery as a major cause of muscle-contraction pain and will be discussed at length in the next chapter.

Musculature of the back—Back muscles are often stiff and weak from too little exercise—a prime target for tension build-up. Make one wrong move with a tense back and you could be in for a lifetime of low-back discomfort.

Cardiovascular—This category includes the heart and *other* muscles connected with the vascular system. Hypertension is the most common expression of stress in this system. Chest pains come in for a close second.

Skin—Psoriasis, eczema, hives: these are all debilitating skin problems that can be precipitated by stress. Less severe skin reactions include flushing and blotching.

Stress-related conditions are not mutually exclusive. In other words, just because you have an ulcer doesn't mean that you can't suffer from headaches too. Not only can you be plagued by several of these disorders, but you can have rotating symptoms. One week you might have a stiff neck that disappears on Tuesday morning only to be replaced by stomach cramps in the afternoon. On Thursday, your stomach feels fine, but you develop a headache, and so on.

These symptoms are the total body's reaction to stress and tension. They act as an offshoot of the body's adaptive capacity to withstand stress. Because the effects of poor adaptive capacity are cumulative, you have to treat them as soon as they appear.

This is especially true of muscle-contraction pain. Muscular discomforts are not just a result of tension. An underlying skeletal imbalance often exists which causes the muscles to remain tense regardless of the emotional climate. Many of us have some skeletal structure that is a little too long or too short, but the muscle strain that the structural imbalance causes doesn't affect us for years. Often these tissues will become sore and painful only when they are further insulted by stress and tension. Stress will always attack the weakest part of your body. Muscles that are already strained because of some skeletal imbalance provide a perfect target.

Structural imbalances, to which we're all prone, often go unnoticed by physicians. One leg's being slightly shorter than the other isn't cause for alarm, but it's a very common imbalance in people with low-back pain. In these cases, no treatment is going to relieve the pain until the leg-length disparity is corrected—with a shoe wedge, for example.

An almost universally unrecognized imbalance in the jaw contributes to muscular pain all over the body. Let's say that you have an unbalanced jaw and a leg-length imbalance, as is common among my patients. Then you suffer from headaches and backaches. If an orthopedist does spot the leg problem and adjusts it, but misses the jaw imbalance, he or she wil not always be able to treat you successfully. On the other hand, if you go to a head-pain specialist who discovers the jaw imbalance but misses the leg problem, he or she won't be able to relieve you completely, either.

Since the whole body works as a unit to combat stress and tension, you have to remove the stress in every part of it in order to relieve discomfort.

Unfortunately, many physicians don't share this approach to chronic pain and other stress-related illness. They will try to attack each symptom or pain in the order of its appearance and reappearance. After a while, however, such doctors may find the recurrence of the symptoms exasperating. Failure to treat your illness successfully may lead your physician to believe that the problem is not medical, but mental. You may be routed to a psychologist or psychiatrist before a holistic approach to your problem is even tried.

Being shuttled from physician to psychologist to specialist and back again often makes the chronic pain victim sicker than he or she was at the start of the treatment. A combination of frustration and mixed or experimental medical treatments would make anyone crazy. After a few years, the standard health-care system may become more of a bane to the chronic pain sufferer than the pain is, not to mention the expense, which in itself creates additional stressful symptoms.

The Chronic Pain Syndrome

Most muscle-tension pain sufferers are psychologically normal. However, if you were to meet some of the patients on their first visit to our office, you probably wouldn't be able to distinguish them from the average *neurotic*, though *functional*, person. The years of pain and frustration they've endured, not to mention being told that they are emotionally unbalanced, has lowered their resistance to daily stress. Weepiness, depression, anxiety—these are all part of a well-documented chain of events in a chronic-pain victim's life. Let's look at what happens.

In the beginning, you may have suffered, say, an occasional headache. You're in your teens. So much else is happening to your body that an occasional headache seems normal.

As the months go by, the headaches get more frequent and more severe. You find that your sleep is interrupted by them. During the day, you're irritable, short-tempered. You don't have a good attention span, and as a result, your work is suffering. The loss of sleep has also affected your appetite. You find that you're never hungry and your stomach upsets easily.

When the pain becomes incapacitating, you see a physician. Obviously, the doctor says, the headaches are tension related. He gives you some codeine and a tranquilizer, and orders some neurological tests just to be sure. When you take the prescribed drugs, they work, but your thought process is slow and fuzzy.

For a while you're pretty anxious about the headaches. Are they going to continue to get worse? How will you be able to lead a normal life with this pain? Will you have to be institutionalized?

You start looking into every possible avenue of treatment. Doctor bills alone can run to $75 a week. And the limitless prescriptions cost $100 a month. But all the tests you take are negative. All the specialists say that the pain isn't serious.

A few more years pass. Your family and friends try to be patient, but most of their sympathy is used up. You have to be picked up from parties when your headache makes it impossible for you to drive. Plans have to be rearranged at the last moment when you're sick. A lot of people, especially dates, are simply not calling anymore.

Whereas you're used to being anxious, you're now depressed. You sleep entire weekends away. Work seems like a herculean task to undertake every day. Desperation wells up. You feel that it's simply not worth the energy to go on.

The psychiatrist prescribes antidepressants. They make you too drowsy to get to work on time. At first you go in late, then not at all. You also start putting on weight. Between the depression, the pain, the weight gain and the empty hours at home, you start thinking about suicide. The family decides to take you back into their house.

After your funds are depleted, the family starts picking up the medical bills. Some of the people from whom you seek help are charlatans. Sometimes you have to take new drugs to counteract the side effects of the old. All these attempts to heal you, or at least to make you stable, cost money. Your family begins to resent the toll of your pain. But your whole life is wrapped up in it.

Who Develops Muscle-Contraction Pain?

The Chronic Pain Syndrome described above is common among pain victims. But what sort of people develop this kind of problem? We haven't been able to discern a prototype. Our patients come to us from all age groups, economic levels, social and cultural backgrounds, and intelligence levels.

In one recent study, we found that 71 percent of a healthy general population of dental patients suffered from chronic pain; of these, 43 percent complained of chronic headaches, 17 percent experienced neckaches, and 11 percent admitted to having both problems. Many of these people were run down by the stresses of urban living, but we found purely behavioral causes of chronic pain as well.

Many people strike and hold unhealthy physical positions when they're working. Housework or maintenance work demands that you be crouched over an iron, a vacuum or a mop for a good part of the day. Unless the muscles that are being abused in these positions are exercised regularly to relax and stretch them, you could develop muscle-contraction pain much like the stress-related disorder. Built-up tension in the muscles causes the same problems whether induced by stress or by physical strain.

In offices, many people abuse the muscles in their heads, necks and shoulders by cupping the phone between the head and shoulder, or propping up the chin on one hand while doing desk work, or absent-mindedly chewing on pens, pencils, pipes or even cigars.

We weren't meant to either hunch over a vacuum or sit at a desk all day, but most of us do one or the other for many years of our adult lives. Without the proper kinds of preventive regimens, anyone—neurotic or level-headed—can easily develop muscle-contraction pain.

What Causes the Pain?

Negative test results don't necessarily mean that no physical cause for your pain exists. Medical tests—even x-rays—can only indicate the presence or absence of some disorders. Muscle spasms, for instance, won't show up in any test. And this is one of the most common causes of chronic pain. Let's look at how muscles cause discomfort.

A healthy muscle contracts when it is in use and relaxes itself when the work is done. Muscles that are affected by stress, however, contract and stay tensed up. After a time in this tense condition, the muscles will go into spasm and be unable to relax at all. If you don't exercise regularly, your body is probably more susceptible to the effects of stress than if you were active. Tension builds up faster in muscles that are weak and stiff from lack of exercise.

When a muscle is always knotted up, blood can't circulate through the tissue to nourish it. Some of the tissue will eventually degenerate and form little nodules called "trigger points." These little knots are a source of much of the severe referred pain associated with muscle-strain problems. Once the pain reference pattern of muscle is known it can be used to locate the muscle that is the source of pain. (See illustrations below*.)

Trigger points can refer pain to other parts of the body far removed from their source. If you have a trigger point in your shoulders, for instance, it could be the cause of the pain in your temple. As a matter of fact, in examining a trigger point in the muscle, you can press it and feel the pain shooting up to the temple. You know, then, that your head pain is actually in the shoulder muscles. On the other hand, if you're unaware of the trigger point, you might mistake the throbbing pain on one side of your head for migraine, a common misdiagnosis.

*Illustrations reproduced from "The Myofascial Genesis of Pain" by Janet Travell and Seymour H. Rinzler, *Postgraduate Medicine* (Vol. 11, No. 5), May 1952.

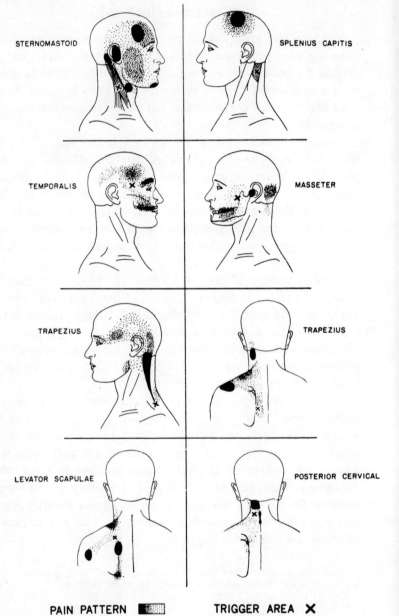

STERNOMASTOID

SPLENIUS CAPITIS

TEMPORALIS

MASSETER

TRAPEZIUS

TRAPEZIUS

LEVATOR SCAPULAE

POSTERIOR CERVICAL

PAIN PATTERN ▨   TRIGGER AREA ✕

SHOULDER AND ARM

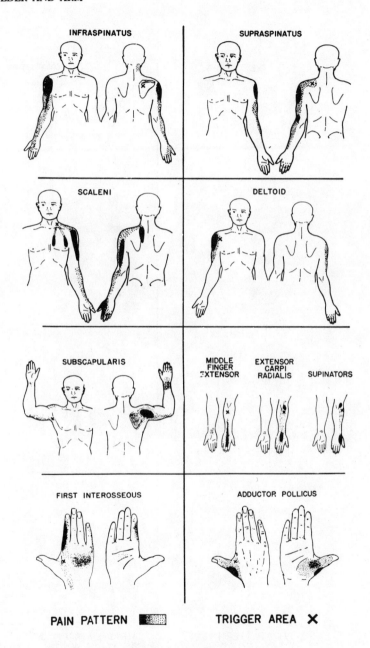

PAIN PATTERN ▮▮▮   TRIGGER AREA ✕

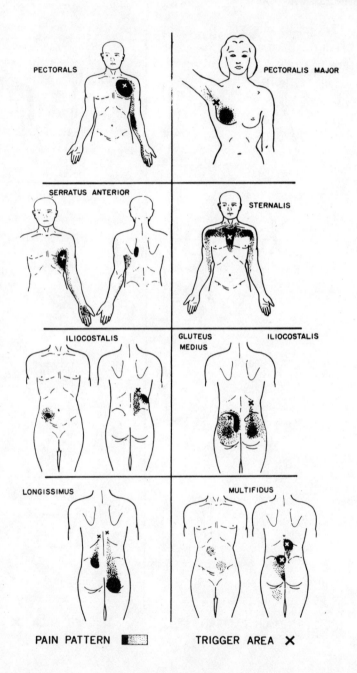

PECTORALS

PECTORALIS MAJOR

SERRATUS ANTERIOR

STERNALIS

ILIOCOSTALIS

GLUTEUS MEDIUS

ILIOCOSTALIS

LONGISSIMUS

MULTIFIDUS

PAIN PATTERN ■

TRIGGER AREA ✗

Trigger points can occur anywhere in the body and cause diagnostic havoc wherever they appear. In the shoulders and neck, they cause pain mistaken for migraine headaches. In the buttocks, the discomfort they bring to the back is often confused with spinal disk disorders. Because they don't show up on conventional diagnostic tests, and because most physicians don't examine the muscles for these trigger points, they are perhaps the greatest factor in the misdiagnosis of chronic muscle-contraction pain. Without proper treatment, these knots continue to cause pain which, in turn, makes you more tense and causes the muscle to contract more tightly, leading to more trigger points and more pain.

The ironic side of this dismal chain of events is that migraines and spinal disk disorders are difficult to treat, while trigger points are easy to dissolve. All that is necessary is that fluid be injected into the knot, or that it be dry-needled. The nodule breaks up and the pain disappears.

The role of trigger points in chronic pain is an important and too often neglected one. In the chapters that follow, I'll explain how these nodules form in the different parts of the body, how they cause pain in the head, neck, back and other areas, and the most frequent misdiagnoses for these muscular pains. But before you go on, I'd like you to read Shirley's story. If you suffer chronic pain, I'm sure you'll empathize with many of her feelings. Although part of her pain is not muscular, we believe that 85 percent of the discomfort is caused by muscle tension.

Shirley

I'm thirty-five and I work as an account executive in an advertising agency. About three years ago, I was in an accident in a cab. I got a concussion and bruised my jaw. The bone seemed to be larger on one side than the other and I was having trouble opening my mouth. Just after the accident I had bad headaches and pain in my neck and upper back too, but my doctors told me that was because of the concussion.

Six months later, I noticed a distinct click in my jaw, aside from the other discomfort. My dentist put a bite plate in my mouth to correct an imbalance that he found. I wore that for a year and a half.

Oh, and I was miserable. All that pain in my head, neck and back. I thought that it couldn't possibly be from the accident any more. It was terrible. I was depressed and anxious all the time. My job suffered. My social life evaporated. I couldn't sleep. I was just a wreck.

So I went the normal route. Saw lots of doctors. Heard over and over how stress was causing all this pain, and took the tranquilizers that were prescribed. Finally, my dentist did another thorough examination and found that my jaw problem had gotten worse.

Shirley is a typical adult pain sufferer. Her whole life had been shattered by the different treatments, the drugs and the hopelessness. But Shirley is still free to keep on searching, to verbalize her frustration, and ultimately to find a specialist who may be able to help her, as we can. Children suffering just as badly are often unable even to tell the doctor what is wrong.

Suffer the Children

Generation after generation, children are brought to physicians complaining of stomach aches, headaches and earaches for which no medical reason can be found. Lawrence Funt, D.D.S., who compiled the chart of chronological TMJ Syndrome symptoms in the next chapter, has studied the manifestations of muscle-spasm pain in all age groups. And his work shows that children, even infants, can suffer the same kinds of muscle-spasm pain syndromes as adults. However, the kinds of chronic pain are different.

The three most common complaints of all children from age four to fourteen are earaches, sore throats and stomach aches. As often as not, these aches exist in the absence of any infection. Stomach aches will come on without nausea or vomiting, and the pain will be just behind the solar plexus rather than down in the stomach.

Physicians are perplexed by these chronic pains which seem to have no cause. They offer antibiotics to stop the development of a yet unseen infection. In three days the child will seem better, but the mother may notice that this is true regardless of the physician's intervention. In three days the earache, sore throat or stomach ache will be relieved. In two weeks the same ailments will reappear in the same mysterious way.

Adolescents from fourteen to seventeen have a different set of symptoms that indicate a chronic muscle-spasm syndrome. These patients complain mostly of stomach ache, with headache and growing pains. The stomach ache is still located behind the solar plexus and still appears to develop without the usual provocation of overeating or illness. The headache always occurs with the stomach ache, or vice versa. It, too, is not connected to any neurological disorders or to infection.

Growing pains in the legs, hips and lower back come and go as mysteriously as the headaches and stomach ailments. These are all common muscle-contraction dysfunctions. Most are caused by some structural imbalance. The children certainly don't know it. Neither do the parents or the doctors. So the children suffer through years of misdiagnosis—perhaps pointing to some psychological disorder— and pain.

We have found that these children don't make up chronic pain. They are rarely hypochondriacs. They are usually not neurotic. And they are not trying to get out of school. Would a child make up an earache that keeps him or her awake and crying all night? Would a child create a stomach ache so severe that he or she clutches the stomach and rolls on the floor in pain? We think not.

In the next chapters, we will discuss where you can go for relief of chronic head, neck and back pain. You should also consider these specialists to rid your children of the chronic pain they may suffer.

2

The TMJ Syndrome and You

If you suffer from headache, neckache, backache or other chronic discomfort, you'll be tested for many diseases and disorders in an attempt to find the cause of the pain. You may be tested for all kinds of obscure afflictions, but ironically, you probably won't be checked for the most common purveyor of pain: the TMJ Syndrome.

TMJ stands for temporomandibular joint, your jaw joint. When these joints are out of alignment, your jaws are unbalanced and you're a prime candidate for the syndrome. This disorder is basically a muscle-contraction or tension problem that initiates head, neck, back and other pain in 80 percent of the chronic-discomfort cases we see today. An estimated 75 million Americans are affected by this syndrome, but it is so often misdiagnosed that only a handful of these people are treated properly.

How the TMJ Syndrome Develops

The TMJ Syndrome begins when the jaw joints are forced out of alignment, causing the upper and lower jaws to meet in an unbalanced relationship. A blow to the head will accomplish this quickly. More often, however, the jaws and the teeth become malpositioned as a result of genetic, nutritional and behavioral factors. Let's look at the role of each of these factors in jaw imbalance.

Genetically speaking, we are far from perfect creations. More than 50 percent of us develop some structural oddity, like one leg shorter than the other, or an irregular tooth-eruption pattern. An irregular tooth-eruption pattern simply means that your teeth will come in crooked, or develop abnormally to some degree. Since the teeth dictate the position of the jaws, misaligned teeth will not properly support the jaws in a balanced position.

Many parents feel that they can ward off future problems arising from irregular tooth positions by having the teeth straightened. Orthodontia may help the teeth meet in a more aesthetic relationship, but often the complicated jaw imbalance persists. The dentist works primarily on tooth-to-tooth relationships. He or she does not always adjust the bite to accommodate an orthopedically correct jaw position. A jaw imbalance, then, might well be reinforced rather than alleviated through various dental procedures.

Nutrition also plays an important part in tooth development. Obviously, if you don't get the proper nourishment as a fetus or while growing up, your teeth won't grow in correctly. Once again, the teeth dictate the position of the jaws, so improperly erupted teeth can cause a jaw imbalance.

Chewing habits are important not only during tooth development, but also in maintaining a proper bite. If you have had a number of teeth pulled because of decay, fractures or unsuccessful root canal therapy, the position of the remaining teeth will change to compensate for the loss, thereby altering the jaw's position.

Many jaw problems result from bad oral habits. Children who suck their thumbs may push the growing teeth out of position. Some learn to swallow so that their tongue pushes the teeth out of line while they're coming in. Others clench and grind their teeth when under stress.

You can see that most of the causes of a jaw imbalance are far more common than a blow to the head or some other kind of accident. Whatever the cause, once a jaw imbalance is created, you are predisposed to developing the TMJ Syndrome later in life.

Stress and the Jaw Imbalance

Once the jaws are unbalanced, your whole body tenses up to share the strain of the imbalance. To understand why the entire body becomes involved in a single joint imbalance, let's look at a function of the jaw other than chewing.

In man, the jaw joints seem to act as the center of body balance. But this is not really an advance over four-legged creatures. Quadrupeds have their weight evenly distributed on four legs, with a tail to balance out the head and body. Their center of balance is about midbody. Man, however, was orthopedically short-changed, having been given no tail and only two legs to walk on. A kind of top-heavy skyscraper was formed. The center of balance moved away from midbody and into the head area in order to keep the skull upright on the meager two-legged support system.

The head, mind you, weighs nine to fourteen pounds, yet it is balanced on only seven cervical or neck vertebrae. That balance is maintained by the lower jaw and its muscles, acting as a counter-weight for the rest of the skull.

Thus, when the jaw is in the proper position, the head rests comfortably on the neck and shoulders. If the lower jaw is forced out of place, however, the head will be thrown off balance and all the muscles supporting it will have to strain to keep it in position on the neck. So all the muscles in the head, neck and shoulders tense up. Then the muscles in the rest of the body are forced to share the stress in and around the head, and they tense up too.

You might think that this tension would be uncomfortable to live with every day. Oddly enough, most people don't notice a thing. One can actually go through life, as many people do, without discomfort from a jaw imbalance. But people who internalize stress or have poor posture and oral habits are easy targets for the TMJ Syndrome.

The syndrome begins when the tense muscles surrounding an imbalanced jaw are further aggravated and go into spasm. For instance, one of the most common precipitators of the TMJ Syndrome is tooth grinding, clenching or gnashing. These are all stress-relieving habits. Most people are unaware that they spend hours with their teeth meshed together. They are also innocent of the trauma that these habits are causing to the muscles in the head, neck, shoulders and back.

People use their jaws for all kinds of stress-releasing habits. There's the jaw jutter, who sets out the jaw in a defiant stance, even when no one is threatening him or her. There's the pencil/pen/ cigar/fingernail chewer, who works away with equal fervor at whatever is placed in the mouth. The nocturnal grinder is a frequent offender, grinding his or her teeth all night, unaware of the damage being done.

Stress, however, is not the only force that leads people to insult the muscles around the jaw joints. Just plain poor posture is another common culprit. Look around you someday when you're watching TV with friends or working at a desk with a number of people. Note how many of them are too tired to hold up their heads. There's always someone in a waiting room or library with his or her chin propped up on a cupped hand. This sign of tiredness, boredom or even attentiveness puts far too much strain on the muscles supporting the jaw.

When already tense muscles are further strained by any of these habits, they go into spasm. The muscles will tighten up so hard that blood won't be able to circulate through them properly. Without sufficient circulation, tissues can't be nourished and one begins to develop those little knots of degenerated tissue—the pain-producing trigger points.

Muscle spasm and trigger points can occur in any part of the body as a result of stress and associated jaw and skeletal imbalance. The pain and other symptoms arising from these spastic muscles make up the TMJ Syndrome. The table at the end of this chapter lists all the body systems that are affected by the syndrome and what kinds of symptoms develop. Common complaints include sharp pains deep behind the eyes and in the temple area, earaches, sinus pain, pain in the jaw joints, intense headaches on one or both sides of the head (commonly mistaken for migraine), or pain in the neck. There may be stiffness in the neck and shoulders, even pain radiating into the arms and hands. Often people complain of sharp shoulder pain and are misdiagnosed as having bursitis. The pain can move down the back and into the legs. The litany of discomfort caused by this syndrome seems endless.

Pain, however, is not the only symptom of the TMJ Syndrome. The unbalanced jaw can create a clicking, grating or crackling sound when you open or close your mouth. Your hearing may be impaired by a constant whooshing or ringing. Some people find that their sinuses are always clogged and their throats sore. Dizziness occurs frequently. Even hormonal imbalances have been connected with the syndrome, as an additional causative factor.

I don't have to tell you that this array of symptoms befuddles a physician who is unacquainted with jaw-imbalance disorders. And most physicians who are familiar with the TMJ Syndrome think of it as a problem that occurs as frequently among their patients as brain tumors. They've also been taught that the symptom to note is pain in the jaw joint. This is only one of many pains a TMJ Syndrome sufferer may have, and it probably won't be the first one mentioned. All the rest of the symptoms I've listed aren't indicative of any one disease. When they occur together, the confused physician may lump them under the nervous-disorder label.

Worse yet, if you complain about a discomfort that can easily be confused with a more recognizable disorder, you could be improperly treated for a disease you don't have. The headache that is so common in TMJ Syndrome is almost universally diagnosed and treated as migraine. Back pains and shooting pain down the legs can lead to a diagnosis of a ruptured disk if the doctor doesn't test for TMJ Syndrome. Standard treatment for a disk problem is surgery.

The backache example is an extreme one. However, many of the complaints caused by a jaw imbalance are improperly treated as psychogenic pain. You'll be provided with tranquilizers and painkillers—sometimes antidepressants. These drugs may seem to make the pain go away at first. They do make you less sensitive to pain, but as your tolerance for the drug increases, the insensitivity to pain decreases. Eventually no amount of medicine will comfort you.

The TMJ Syndrome's pain can be relieved in only one way: The jaw has to be repositioned properly. When this simple procedure is done, your muscles can finally relax. No medications or operations can help the pain, because they don't take away the cause—the skeletal imbalance that is straining the muscles.

Let's look at a particular type case of TMJ Syndrome. You're thirteen years old and have worn braces. The teeth take about three years to straighten out. By the time you're ready for college, your bite is considered perfect. Yet you notice a clicking whenever you open or close your mouth. You never noticed that sound before the braces were fitted.

In college, you go through your first exam period. Every morning you wake up with sore, tired jaws. Subconsciously, you've been working off your tension by grinding your teeth at night. When exams are over, however, the soreness goes away and you don't think about it anymore.

Now you've graduated and found a job. The pressure's really on. You find that whenever you sit back for a breather, you practically have to unlatch your jaws because the teeth are clenched so tightly.

A few months pass and you notice that you're getting headaches almost every day. First they come on at the end of the day and get worse until bedtime. Later on, they are present from the time you wake until you go to sleep. Steadily they increase in severity until you have to take a leave of absence from work.

In this case, the jaw imbalance was created by the improper tooth positions prior to as well as following orthodontic therapy. Later, the already tense muscles around the jaw were abused further by tooth clenching. The muscles went into spasm. Trigger points developed. And you ended up with one of the most common symptoms of the TMJ Syndrome: severe headache.

Unfortunately, you probably won't guess that your problem is physical. You'll feel incompetent, a victim of your emotions. You'll wonder why you're not capable of handling the normal pressures of adult life. These feelings of anxiety regarding the pain will probably trigger the Chronic Pain Syndrome discussed in Chapter 1. The Chronic Pain Syndrome will put you under more stress and cause more severe symptoms of the TMJ Syndrome. The vicious cycle begins.

Of course, there are many variations on this theme. Some people develop symptoms as early as age four. Some never feel a thing until they're sixty. We have found, though, that the effects of a jaw imbalance are cumulative. If you have a jaw imbalance for two years, the symptoms of the syndrome will reflect the trauma suffered by the muscles for two years. If you have a jaw imbalance for twenty-five years before the syndrome appears, your symptoms will reflect twenty-five years of muscle strain.

Growing Up with the TMJ Syndrome

For a long time, we couldn't find a pattern in the symptoms of the TMJ Syndrome. There seemed to be no limit or order to the discomforts that arose when the jaw was out of balance. However, in recent years, as more cases of the syndrome were recognized and treated, a chronological pattern emerged. You could see the progression of the disease from the patterns of symptoms in different age groups.

Rather than give you just the chronological chart of symptoms, Doctors Funt and Stack, both TMJ specialists from the Washington, D.C., area, decided to let people in the different age groups speak for themselves. In each group we found one person who was the most characteristic of his or her stage of the syndrome. That person wrote down in his or her own words the feelings and discomforts being experienced. In addition, we compiled a composite patient who represents the person most frequently seen with this disorder.

After familiarizing yourself with these descriptions, you should be able to recognize key symptoms of a jaw disorder. Later on in this chapter, I'll suggest some other methods of determining whether or not you have the TMJ Syndrome.

The Composite Patient

"I'm twenty-five to thirty-five years of age and really don't know what is happening to me. Oh, yes, I've had headaches, but they now seem to be getting worse. There are times when the headaches are so bad that I vomit. Other times, it feels like a spike is being driven through the top of my head. My friends joke with me about drinking too much because my eyes are bloodshot when I come in to work. I must admit my eyes do hurt—not up front, where they're bloodshot, but deep behind. I feel kind of foolish mentioning this, but I have a roaring noise in my left ear. Sometimes it is so loud that it masks out the street sounds. Lately when I get up in the morning, I'm sort of dizzy. It's not like the room is spinning around me, but more like me spinning. Sometimes after getting up, I have to lean on the wall till things straighten out. I've gone to my orthopedist because of the pains in my neck and bursitis in my left shoulder. He said the only thing that seems unusual is the curvature of my spine, and that couldn't be a reason for my neck and shoulder problems."

Susan (ages 4–7)

Susan has had colds and bouts with the flu. She has also had the usual ear infections and occasionally tonsillitis. She is no different than hundreds of thousands of other four-year-olds except that she has headaches around her forehead and in her temples. She's had them for so long that it's just a part of her everyday life. By age 5, she is able to communicate with more people her age (in kindergarten), and her friends on occasion will ask the school nurse for aspirin for what they call "headache." Susan has had stomach aches, toothaches and backaches, and her joints would ache when she had the flu, but she really doesn't know what her friends mean by "headaches."

By age 6 to 7, Susan began to notice a feeling of numbness in her forehead and/or temple areas when her mother gave her aspirin for a fever. This didn't happen every time she took aspirin, just sometimes. The "numbness" she experienced was a strange feeling at

first, but in time she felt better when she had "that numbness."
Susan was also having homework, and her eyes would hurt (eye
strain); sinusitis was also a culprit to contend with. Susan found that
aspirin did indeed help the pain of her sinus problem, and sometimes she had that feeling of numbness in her head, and sometimes
she didn't.

Susan is having two different kinds of headaches: muscle-
contraction headaches, on which aspirin has no effect (the kind of
headaches caused by the TMJ Syndrome), and the headaches
stemming from stress, indigestion and fever. She is beginning to
realize that the "numbness" she has experienced is the absence of
what is called pain.

Susan's best friend, Margaret Jones, has "earaches" almost all
the time. Her pediatrician is really frustrated because sometimes
Margaret's ear or ears are infected, but most times they are not, yet
the "earaches" persist. Mrs. Jones is always after Margaret to keep
her mouth closed. The pediatrician can see no nasal blockage, and
so Margaret just has "bad manners." Margaret has told Susan that
the ache in her ears is a little more bearable if she holds her mouth
open, and as a matter of fact, the ache is lots better when Margaret
has a "nose cold" and she has to breathe through her mouth.

Susan and Margaret both suffer from the TMJ Syndrome

Janet (ages 8–10)

Janet has been sent home from school again. Her teacher and
principal are concerned because Janet's grades are not as good as
they have been, and her attention span has diminished. Janet's
mother has noticed that Janet is getting "antsy" at home as well as
in school. Janet's head hurts most of the time now. It is hard for her
to concentrate on her homework, and while at school she feels very
edgy. She would like to leave her desk and just walk around. The
schoolroom is confining. She is not bad; just nervous. Sleeping is
also a problem. Janet wakes frequently during the night and is
therefore not at all rested when the alarm goes off at 7 A.M.

Janet feels badly enough about her teacher's disappointment with her grades, but she also feels sad because she finds herself snapping at her parents over minuscule things. Janet's physician has examined her and can give no reason for her head pains other than a history of "migraine" in the family. The neck soreness that Janet is becoming more aware of also can't be explained. Sometimes the soreness seems to go up her neck to the back of her head. There are also periods of ringing in her ears. Her hearing is normal. But Janet does have unbalanced jaws.

Carol (ages 11–15)

Carol has always complained of headache and pain in her sinus cavities—"just like her mother," everyone said. Carol's face feels tired when she wakes up, and as the day wears on, her jaws are positively weak. Chewing hard or tough food hurts, so she went with her mother to their dentist. The dentist carefully examined Carol's teeth, but could find nothing wrong with them. Her teeth did show some wear from grinding them, but most people grind their teeth—some more, some less. The dentist suggested that Carol might be a little nervous and that perhaps a mild tranquilizer might be considered.

Carol was a determined young lady, and by really concentrating, she was able to do well at school and have pleasant relationships with her friends even though she suffered from almost incessant earaches, eye pain, and annoying grinding and popping noises in her jaw joint. Carol, of course, is a victim of the TMJ Syndrome.

Henry (ages 15–20)

Henry did very well in high school, so it was difficult to understand why he was coming home from college in the middle of his sophomore year. Henry says, "I feel like an old man. I am just so tired all the time that I'm drained of enthusiasm and optimism. Things just aren't exciting anymore." Henry's physician suggested that he see a psychiatrist, since he was anxious and mildly depressed. The psychiatrist agreed with the diagnosis of the physician, but Henry confided to the psychiatrist that he just couldn't deal with the pressure of college. "Why, there were times when I would find myself clenching my teeth, and I wasn't even mad at anyone," Henry said.

At Henry's six-month dental examination, his dentist mentioned the fact that Henry's teeth were showing signs of extreme wear for a nineteen-year-old. "I didn't even tell the dentist that some mornings I couldn't open my jaw very far. As the day wears on, the jaw sort of loosens up and gets better, so I didn't think it was important." Of course it is important—Henry's jaw is unbalanced.

George (ages 20–30)

George has finished his residency in surgery and has been in practice for two years. He is a busy surgeon, on the go all the time. "I could deal with my migraines because they gave notice of their onset and with proper medication could be intercepted most of the time, but not always. My 'other' headaches were not only increasing in intensity, but are now occurring four or five times a week." Aspirin, Valium, codeine, Demerol and now Percodan are on George's list of pain drugs—all to little or no avail, because they do nothing about the position of his jaw.

Jo-Anne (ages 31–40)

"I'm married to a wonderful armed forces officer and have two very active children. I've been in the hospital for two weeks now. The doctors have done just about everything to help me, but there's no letup of the pain in my face and head. I've been fighting the pain for seven years. The doctors want to discharge me, but I will not leave the hospital. I can't go home—I'm desperate from the pain and I am afraid to trust myself alone at home. If it weren't for my husband and children, I'd leave this life of pain."

Mary (ages 41–50)

"All my symptoms over the years have progressively gotten worse. My dentist has just informed me that his routine x-ray exam indicates that part of my jaw joint on the left side is breaking down. He says it must be related to an arthritic condition, yet I don't have arthritis anywhere else.''

Carl (ages 51–60)

"I've lost a lot of teeth over the years. It started with a back molar that hurt. My doctor tested the tooth, and it tested normal. The pain persisted, and the tooth had the nerve taken out of it to stop the pain. The pain continued and it seemed to involve the next molar. The same procedure was followed. I've had three molars removed, including the teeth in front of the back molars, and still the pain continues.''

Marion (ages 61–70)

"I must be just plain wearing out. You'd think by now that I'd be done with all the patching and sewing necessary to keep a body together. I've been in the hospital for two weeks now and without a minute's rest. My jaw, lips and tongue are just moving and wandering all the time. The doctors say the muscles of my face and tongue and jaws have lost all sense of space and just wander without real control. The hospital dentists were called in also. They're just as baffled as the physicians. I guess it really isn't a dental problem, because I don't have any teeth.''

Jo-Anne, Mary, Carl and Marion all exhibit the last stages of the TMJ Syndrome. The battle, in their cases, has been lost.

How to Recognize the TMJ Syndrome

You probably can't make a definite diagnosis for yourself of one disease or another. However, enough indications of a jaw imbalance are easily discernible for you to confirm a suspicion. Here are some signs to look for:

Tired or sore jaws

If you wake up with sore jaws that are difficult and painful to open, start checking yourself occasionally to see if you're subconsciously grinding or clenching your teeth. Chances are that if you clench or grind them during the day, you do the same at night.

Crackling or clicking noises when the jaw moves

Aside from hearing these noises, you can actually feel the click. Put your two small fingers in your ears and press forward lightly. Then open and close your mouth. If your jaws are unbalanced, you'll feel the click. Testing for the click can also be done with the fingers pressing against the joint just outside the ear, as you can see in the illustrations here.

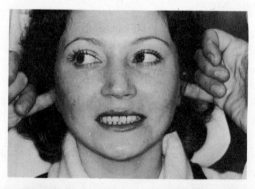

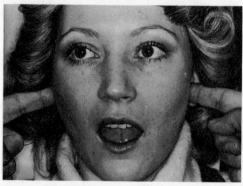

Ringing or whooshing sounds in the ears

Most people are embarrassed to point out this symptom at all.
After all, if you're suffering chronic pain and hearing noises too,
you must be crazy, right? Well, you can put your mind at ease,
because this is a common sign of the TMJ Syndrome.

Feature imbalance

This is one of the most definitive indications of a jaw imbalance.
Often by just looking at a person's face, you can tell on which side
the jaw is unbalanced, as well as on which side the pain is
developing.

Stand in front of a full-length mirror so that you can check for
imbalances down the whole body. Look at your face. Is one eye

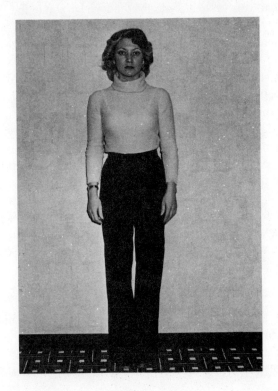

higher and larger than the other? Are your lips turned up on the side of the higher eye? Is the ear on that side higher than the other ear?

If your answer to these questions was yes, you probably have a jaw imbalance on the side of your face where the features are higher.

If you continue down the body, you'll find that the level of the shoulders, breasts and hips are lower on the side where the facial features are higher. The leg on this side is usually shorter than the other too.

By just looking in the mirror, then, you can not only find some fairly sure indications of a jaw imbalance, but you can also see how such an imbalance causes changes in the whole posture of the body.

Treating the TMJ Syndrome

Now that you've heard all the bad news about the TMJ Syndrome, I'll tell you the good. It's easy to treat. The real problem up to this point has been in misdiagnosis, not in inability to treat this disorder.

Usually the program has four phases: (1) relief of pain; (2) correction of jaw imbalance; (3) therapy for poor oral habits; (4) strategies for coping more effectively with stress.

The TMJ Syndrome demands the attention of a dentist. Your physician may be able to treat the muscles and help you with relaxation exercises, but a dentist is the only medical professional who knows how to position the jaws properly.

The first step in treating the TMJ Syndrome, as in treating any other chronic pain, is to relieve the pain. When the hurt is gone, you are less anxious. You sleep and eat better. And because you feel better, you respond to the rest of the treatment more quickly.

Therapy for muscles and trigger points

Muscles and trigger points are the main targets in the earliest part of the treatment, since they are causing the pain. Spastic muscles are coaxed into relaxing with warm as well as cold packs.

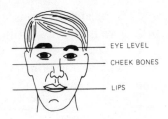

Warmth increases local circulation and reduces muscle tension. Used four times a day for fifteen to twenty minutes, a heating pad or some other form of applied heat will relax strained muscles and soothe the soreness.

In some cases, cold packs are more effective than hot ones. Usually you have to try both to find out which works better for you. Cold seems to lower tissue sensitivity and lessen pain intensity. In the absence of pain, the muscle will relax and the discomfort will disappear.

Topical anesthetics are available that effectively freeze out pain. These obviate leaving whatever you're doing to lie down for a half hour as you must when using a cold compress. An anesthetic such as Fluori-Methane or ethyl chloride spray applied to the painful muscle can ward off a muscle-contraction headache. The pain sensation will be reduced, the muscle will relax, and the headache will be aborted. Yet these anesthetics, unlike painkilling drugs, don't circulate in the body, don't cause side effects or dependence, and so are safe to use and difficult to abuse.

Some of the pain-reducing instruments we use in the office are based on ultrasound and electrical stimulation. Application of ultrasound to a muscle produces heat deep within the tissues. The blood circulates better in the muscle and it begins to relax.

Electrical stimulation causes much the same effects as ultrasound therapy. We use an electrogalvanic stimulator, an increasingly popular method of reducing pain in all kinds of muscular disorders. With this device, a current is passed through the muscle, creating no discomfort in you, but sufficiently exciting the tissue to increase blood circulation, cause relaxation and increase flexibility. Using the current in conjunction with careful exercise, you can be relieved of headaches, neck pains, even backaches in fifteen minutes.

A new addition to electrical pain relief is the transcutaneous nerve stimulator. This device works on the principle that electricity not only can increase circulation and muscle relaxation, but can actually scramble the nerve's pain message to the brain, and increase the production of pain-relieving substances.

Lastly in our muscle-relaxing efforts, we use old-fashioned massage. Gentle rubbing of the muscles around the face and head can help them relax. With the shoulder and neck muscles, more vigorous massage is used.

Relaxing the spastic muscles is one step toward eliminating discomfort. But these methods are often ineffective against trigger points deep within the tissue. Trigger points have to be broken up either by fluid injection or by dry needling. Since they are the source of much of the acute pain you might suffer, trigger points have to be treated along with tense muscles to truly eliminate pain.

We've seen people who were literally crippled with pain become completely symptom-free after one diligent application of muscle-relaxation and trigger-point therapy. But they won't remain that way unless their jaw balance is restored, because the unbalanced jaw will initiate all over again the whole sequence of strained muscles going into spasm and developing trigger points.

Correcting the jaw imbalance

For the trained dentist, correcting the bite is not a complicated procedure. It is necessary to discover where and how the jaw is unbalanced and then judge how to reposition the teeth to support the jaw properly. Changing the way your teeth meet—in other words, your bite—is accomplished with a removable acrylic bite appliance for the upper or lower teeth.

While you can remove the appliance to clean it, there is usually no other reason to take it out. The appliance is ground down to approximate the shape of the teeth it is covering, so you can chew as easily with the appliance as without it. Most people have no difficulty talking, eating or sleeping with the appliance in their mouth.

As therapy continues and your muscles relax, the position of the jaw might change every three weeks or so. The attending dentist will accommodate the shift in the jaw balance by grinding down or building up the appliance to adjust your bite. After several months, the position of the jaw and your bite will be stable. Only at this point will arrangements be made to alter your bite permanently in order to support the jaws in their proper position. This alteration can be accomplished with caps, heightened fillings, removable oral appliances or orthodontic therapy.

At the end of this part of the treatment, pain and other symptoms will be gone and the imbalance that caused the muscles to go into spasm will have been adjusted. However, if you go back to your old habits of tooth grinding, pen chewing or chin propping, you could end up in the same trouble a few years down the road. The last two steps in therapy will prevent that from happening.

Changing oral habits

Our exercises are designed to help restore the proper tone and elasticity of the muscles in the head and neck to eliminate tooth clenching and grinding behavior, and to teach you the proper way of opening and closing the mouth.

The first and easiest exercise is a simple stretching of the jaw muscles. You open your mouth wide and then close it in a rhythmic, hingelike movement. This helps restore full movement of the jaw, which is often lost when the TMJ Syndrome develops.

A second stretching exercise is aimed at teaching you how to open your mouth without protruding the lower jaw. Most people arch out the lower jaw when they talk or eat, which often causes the click common to the TMJ Syndrome. The jaw was meant to work as a hinge—lowered down and back. When it is arched out every time the mouth is opened, it is being forced out of its proper position. This, of course, leads to muscle strain.

In this second exercise, you curl up your tongue and place it as far back on the roof of the mouth as possible. With the tongue locked in that position, open and close your mouth. Keeping the tongue on the roof of the mouth limits the movement of your jaw to a down and back swing. By repeating this exercise, you relearn how to use your jaws.

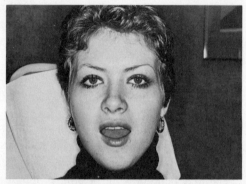

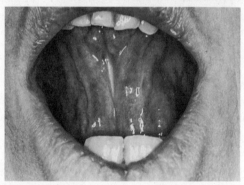

Finally, we have an exercise to relax the jaw muscles. Much like the first jaw-stretch muscle toner, the stretch-against-resistance muscle relaxer requires you only to open and close the mouth. But in this exercise, the jaw rests on one fist. Your hand provides the resistance against which to exercise. Using an opposing force in exercise has a relaxing effect on the muscles.

After each stretch-against-resistance exercise set, you return to the plain stretching exercises for one set. This helps stretch and tone the muscles when they're in a relaxed state. Other exercises used in therapy are explained in the Corrective Exercises section at the end of this chapter.

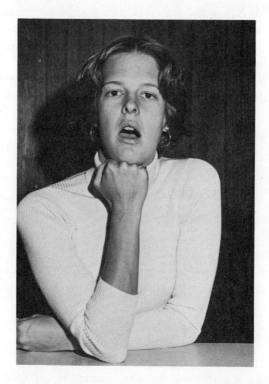

The physical exercises work together with a mental suggestion to prevent you from further abusing the muscles in your head and neck. We instruct not only the patients but their family and friends, as well as the staff, to repeat to themselves: "Lips together, teeth apart." Most people are unaware that the teeth are not supposed to be touching except when you swallow. Keeping the teeth together when they're not in use is the first step to clenching and grinding. If you repeat this little phrase to yourself as often as possible, you'll notice that your bad oral habits will begin to diminish. If you're consciously keeping your teeth apart, how can you subconsciously grind them?

Coping with Stress

Most TMJ Syndrome sufferers cope poorly with stress. We have found, however, that training with biofeedback, relaxation exercises and/or self-hypnosis, as well as instituting a stress-reducing diet, can eventually increase a person's capacity for stress.

Biofeedback, relaxation exercises, self-hypnosis and the diet can and should be used at home. To that end, we've provided two chapters in this book to help you start your own regimen. One deals with nutrition, and the other outlines different kinds of tension-relieving exercises.

TMJ Sufferers Speak for Themselves

All of these ideas about jaw imbalance as a predominant cause of chronic muscle-tension pain are probably new to you. But if you listen to how it has affected many patients, and how they found relief, you'll see how very common the symptoms of the TMJ Syndrome are. Here, then, are three relieved chronic-pain sufferers to tell their stories:

Bunny

"My story is a little odd because I made the same mistake twice. About three years ago, I had a terrible infection in my ears. It started in the left and spread to the right and down into my sinuses. From that time on, my sinuses were very susceptible to infection.

"At that time, I was also being treated by a chiropractor for neck and back pain, with which I'd suffered for years. So while I was a healthy person in general, I did suffer these two chronic disorders.

"Then, just after the ear infection subsided, I began to develop these unusual head pains. I'd never felt anything like them before. The pain went around my forehead, into the jaw joints and cheeks, and eventually all over my head, scalp, in my ears and neck. I couldn't lie down in any position. I couldn't put my head on a pillow, no matter how lightly, without feeling this excruciating pain. So I couldn't get any rest. I tried sleeping in a sitting position, but if I leaned my head back, the pain would be unbearable.

"I was really incapacitated. I had to rest during the day because I didn't get enough sleep at night. And I was depressed. When I had to go somewhere, I felt so badly during the period I was out driving or visiting or having dinner with people that it was unbearable. I could hardly speak because even talking made the pain worse.

"I'm not one to run quickly to doctors, but I started seeing every specialist I could think of to help me. I was seeing the chiropractor, sinus specialists, ear specialists and allergy doctors. Sometimes I would get a prescription for painkillers, but no one could find the cause of my headaches. The doctors didn't really have any explanation. That was so defeating and frustrating. I was on a merry-go-round of chasing to doctors, one after another. Every day I went to a new one, hoping in vain for them at least to tell me what the problem was, so we'd know whether or not it was treatable. That was what made me very depressed, because nobody knew, nobody could say what was wrong.

"Finally, my chiropractor referred me to a dentist who specialized in jaw disorders. It had never dawned on me that the problem could be in my mouth. But this dentist took one look at me and knew exactly what was wrong—the TMJ Syndrome.

"I was given a temporary appliance to wear that would correct my bite and the jaw imbalance. Sure enough, the headaches gradually went away and I experienced definite relief in my neck and back as well.

"That was about two years ago. For all this time, I was feeling fine. I wore my appliance religiously. But suddenly my headaches started coming back. And again I thought that it had to be a sinus problem or an allergy to something. So I started on the same medical merry-go-round, being told that there was no problem anywhere in my head that could cause the pain.

"Along with the headaches came the neck pain. And finally, after I'd been told countless times that there was no infection or other organic problem in my head, it occurred to me that something might be wrong with the bite plate. I went back to the dentist. He built up my plate. The next day, I was free of the pain in my neck, head and ears. That's the miracle. That's the incredibility of the whole thing. It's the closest thing to magic I've seen in my whole life."

Mildred

"I'm thirty-three years old and a social worker. I've had pain in my back since I was seventeen. I don't know what really caused the first attack. I seem to remember doing some exercises like leg lifts and sit-ups. Anyway, I awoke one morning, got up to go to the bathroom, and almost passed out from the pain in my back. I couldn't walk or sit. For a couple of weeks I was like that, totally dependent on other people to get me things. And I was supposed to be leaving for college—to live on my own for the first time.

"We went to an orthopedist who was a friend of the family. He basically told me to stay in bed until the pain passed and to wear a corset thereafter. Then he gave me a set of exercises to strengthen my back. I went to college with the corset. It was horrendous. I didn't wear it very much because it always caused me more discomfort than it was worth.

"The pain, however, did go away and I was fine for a number of years. Oh, periodically I'd do something too strenuous and my back would be thrown out again, but nothing like that first time. I've really only had two or three incidents like that one. Like the time three years ago when I was putting up a towel rack. I was obviously leaning over in a way that gave no support to my back muscles. It went into spasm immediately and I was in bed for a few days. You do absolutely nothing and it just goes.

"So during my twenties, I basically treated myself. I decided that the answer for me was to exercise and keep my body in good shape. I think now that in some ways I caused more problems than I did good because of the kinds of exercise that I did. My basic philosophy was that I wasn't going to accept this and I was going to plunge ahead as though nothing were wrong. In the course of doing this, I would build up my muscles and be fine.

"In the last year or so, at least one of the exercise regimens, which included a headstand, caught up with me. I started to have difficulty higher up in my back and neck. I'd get stiffness and pain in both those areas. Sometimes it would feel dull and lingering, other times it would be sharp. I couldn't move my neck and I was just miserable.

"I finally decided to see this chiropractor who had been recommended to me. He told me that the course of treatment for my problem would take nine months to a year and would involve heat treatment, manipulation, sonar treatment and exercise. I would have to see him two or three times a week for a year. It sounded horrendous to me. I didn't want to spend my life sitting in a doctor's office.

"Finally, I found a chiropractor who was seeing people six to eight times and really helping. He told me immediately that he felt I had the TMJ Syndrome and that he'd do what he could, but I'd probably have to have my jaw fixed.

"After six visits, there was improvement, but it wasn't lasting, so the chiropractor referred me to a TMJ specialist. Since I started this treatment, I feel much less pain in my neck and back. I have a greater ability to move my neck. Also, the biofeedback training has had a tremendous impact on how I deal with everyday life.

"Of course, I still have some discomfort. There's a lot of tension in my neck still. But with the biofeedback exercises, I can identify the tense muscles and release it. I have control.

"It's hard to say how this has affected my life. Certain incidents come to mind. For instance, I play the piano. When I used to practice, after fifteen or twenty minutes I'd have a pain on the right side of my spine that was so uncomfortable I'd have to stop and lie down on the floor. Then I'd have to exercise to relieve the muscle spasm. I don't have that problem anymore."

Sheila

"I'm twenty-four and have had headaches since high school, I think. It's hard to tell, really, because I thought it was normal to have headaches, so I never paid much attention to them. I thought you got them from driving, reading too much, doing anything for a long time, or when you're under pressure. I guess I'm performance oriented. I work for an advertising agency and I'm always under a lot of strain.

"The headaches were never that bad until I got this jaw problem. I opened my mouth too wide one day and pulled the jaw out. The next morning, it hurt a lot and I couldn't open my mouth very wide. I really didn't connect how bad my headache was with my pulled jaw, even though it got much worse at that time. And there was this terrible click in one side of my jaw whenever I opened or closed my mouth.

"I went to a dentist who specialized in jaw problems and he told me that my problem was not only from opening my mouth too wide, but also from stress. He prescribed Valium and Librium and constructed a bite plate for my mouth. The appliance was for the top of my mouth. Everyone could see it, so wearing the mouthpiece was embarrassing. Aside from that, I wasn't getting much better. That terrible click was still there, I couldn't open my mouth comfortably, and I still had the headaches.

"After seeing that dentist for two months, I moved and was referred to another specialist. This dentist explained the jaw imbalance to me and how he would treat it. He explained why the old appliance hadn't worked and had a new one made. Then he asked, 'Do you get headaches?' I said, 'Yeah, doesn't everybody?' He said, 'No; it's because your jaw is out of balance. I can help you.'

"So I went in for treatment. I remember I walked in there the first morning and said 'I've got another headache.' It was a bad one. I'd get them sometimes in the morning. But I also started having headaches anytime during the day. It was ridiculous. Anyway, he put the new appliance in my mouth and said, 'Now I'll get rid of your headache.' I said, 'Sure.' Well, ten minutes after he'd adjusted the new mouthpiece, the headache was gone. I didn't get another headache for six months. It was amazing. And the cracking was gone too.

"Now my jaw is back to normal and I don't get headaches except when I really push myself too hard. To wake up in the morning without a headache, and to go to bed without one, without using drugs—that's really nice."

Symptoms Associated with the TMJ Syndrome*

Jaw, ear, head and neck symptoms

Jaw—clicking and creaking noises on opening and closing the mouth; upper and lower jaw have too extensive a range of movement on opening and can lock open forward of joint; pain or tenderness of the jaw joint; numbness of and around the teeth; limited ability to open and close mouth; pain in teeth mimicking toothache; evidence of clenching or grinding teeth such as worn areas on teeth; gum disease, dry mouth, burning sensation on tongue and in mouth; puffy and distended lips; ropy saliva; calculus deposits
Ear—excess wax in ears; itching; subjective ear noises; earaches; dizziness; sensation of falling; conductive hearing loss
Head and neck—headache, including migraine; sensitive scalp; neuralgic pains; ache and tiredness in nape of neck and shoulders

Respiratory symptoms

Sinus and throat—postnasal drip; habitual clearing of throat; sinusitis; chronic colds; laryngitis; chronic sore throat or tonsillitis; sneezing; hay fever; asthma

Eye symptoms

inflammation; inflammation of the iris; sensitivity to light; blurred vision; itching; burning; tearing; muscle twitching below the eye

Skin and hair symptoms

Skin—dry; chronic rashes; dermatitis; acne
Hair—dry and brittle; hair loss

*From *The Dental Physician.* Blacksburg, Virginia: Aelred C. Fonder University Publications, 1977.

Gastrointestinal symptoms

upset stomach; heartburn; gas; nausea; constipation; diarrhea; bladder infections; kidney infections

Gynecological symptoms

irregular menstrual cycle; premenstrual tension; premenstrual or midmenstrual cramps and pain; excessive menstrual flow; amenorrhea; frigidity; history of miscarriages or inability to conceive

General symptoms

chronic tiredness; increased nervous tension; malaise; restless sleep; numbness of hands; cold hands and feet; back and leg aches; thirst; lowered hemoglobin in blood; lowered thyroid activity

Mental symptoms

depression; irritation; worry; melancholia; hypochondria; excessive nightmares; forgetfulness

Body-posture problems

curvature of the spine and other spinal irregularities; uneven shoulder height; head tilted toward elevated shoulder; pelvis rotated forward on one side; uneven leg length; rounding of shoulders.

The TMJ Syndrome Symptoms:
Chronological Sequence*

Ages 4–7   headaches; stuffiness and/or itching in the ears; earaches with no infection; grinding or clenching the teeth

*From Funt-Stack Index of the Craniomandibular Pain Syndrome

Ages 8–10   headaches; ringing sounds in the ears; back teeth sore; popping or clicking sound when mouth is opened or closed

Ages 11–15   headaches; bloodshot eyes; curvature of the spine; roaring, buzzing and hissing sounds in the ears; dizziness; muscles surrounding jaw joints sore; back teeth sore; creaking sound when mouth is opened or closed; limited ability to open mouth

Ages 16–20   headaches; pain behind the eyes; neck and shoulder pain; curvature of the spine; roaring and ringing sounds in the ears; dizziness; back teeth painful; jaw joints painful to move

Ages 21–30   headaches; frequent sinuslike pain; facial features asymmetrical; pain behind the eyes; neck and shoulder pain; backaches; facial pains; muscles surrounding jaws sore and tired

Ages 31–40   severe headaches; pain behind the eyes; chronic sore throat; shoulder pain mimicking bursitis; numbness in the arms; neck pains; backaches; facial pains; jaw joint becoming arthritic

Ages 41–50   severe headaches; severe pain behind the eyes; numbness in the arms; incapacitating neck pain; incapacitating facial pain; osteoarthritic degeneration of the jaw joint

Ages 51–60   compounding of almost all the previously mentioned symptoms

Ages 61–70   loss of control over movement in face, tongue and lips; other associated symptoms

Corrective Exercises*

Preliminary exercise—Shoulder shrug: Shoulders are brought up as if trying to touch the ears, and then dropped. This exercise can be

---

*Courtesy of Yale Palchick, D.D.S., Akron, Ohio.

used throughout the day to relax and stretch neck and shoulder muscles. It should always precede the following exercise routine.

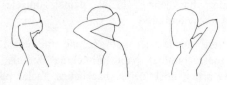

1. Clasp your fingers behind your head. Gently, with a slight amount of resistance, pull your elbows forward until they touch together in front. Then allow your fingers to slide apart and bring elbows as far back as possible. Do this twice in each of two exercise sessions a day.

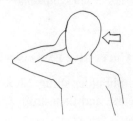

2. Push your hand down on a scale to establish how much pressure is equal to five pounds. Using no more than five pounds of hand resistance against your head, bend it to the right as far as possible, then bring it back up to an upright position. Follow the same procedure through to the left, forward and backward. Make your movements in this exercise gradual and fluid; don't just drop your head one way or the other. Once you've reached the farthest bending position, immediately start bringing your head back to the resting position.

3. Let your jaw hang loose. Bend over as far as possible and clasp your hands together in front of you with arms outstretched. Rise to an upright position, bringing your hands up and above your head. Then break hands apart and continue to make a big circle. Conclude by bending slightly forward and dangling your arms.

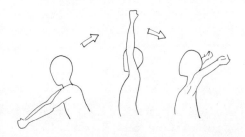

4. Put your hands on your shoulders, keeping elbows together in front of you. Move elbows upward until you have to break them apart. Then continue rotating them in a circle. When arms are even with sides, slip fingers off shoulders and extend arms backward while bending forward. This exercise should end with arms dangling and should be done only once during the two daily exercise sessions at the beginning of your treatment program. Gradually increase the repetition as your treatment proceeds.

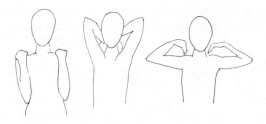

5. Raise arms out to the side. Rotate arms in one-foot circles ten times in one direction, then ten times in the other.

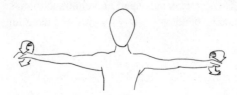

6. Place hand on right side of jaw. Push jaw against the hand, using five pounds of resistance. Repeat to the left. Do once, two times a day, gradually increasing repetition as treatment progresses.

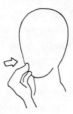

7. Place flat of hand on your forehead and push head forward against it, using five pounds of resistance. Do this once, two times daily. Increase repetitions as treatment progresses.

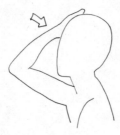

8. Place flat of hand on lower back of head. Push head back, using five pounds of resistance. Do this once, twice a day, increasing repetition as treatment progresses.

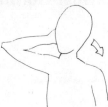

9. Place flat of hand against temple and push against the hand, using five pounds of resistance. Repeat on both left and right sides. This exercise should also be done once, twice a day, gradually increasing the repetitions as treatment progresses.

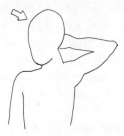

10. Raggedy Ann: Standing erect, bend forward from the waist as far as possible. Alternately raise one shoulder and lower the other. Repeat five to ten times. (If possible, women patients should do this exercise without a bra.)

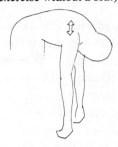

3

Headache: The Most Common Complaint

Forty-two million Americans suffer from chronic headaches. Turn on the TV any night and you'll see the most common kinds of head pain illustrated in ads for aspirin and aspirin substitutes: the throbbing red light on one side of the head; the vise clamping around the top of the head; the slow spread of pain from the neck muscles up and around the head. Unfortunately, the products advertised in these commercials provide little lasting relief for most chronic headaches. We have a treatment, however, which requires no painkillers and works 85 percent of the time for the majority of headache sufferers.

Our research shows that nine out of ten of those throbbing, dull, continuous headaches are caused by muscle contraction or tension. Seventy-five percent of all muscular headaches seem to be precipitated by the TMJ—or jaw-joint—Syndrome, which we discussed in Chapter 3. If you treat the jaw, the headaches will disappear forever.

Muscle-contraction headaches may be the most common kind of head pain, but they are by no means the most severe. Vascular headaches—or "sick headaches," as many sufferers call them—which often appear as a blinding pain on one side of the head, are far more painful than muscular headaches. Though we still lack an absolute definition of the cause of vascular pain, and consequently, a method of treating it, we have found ways of lessening the intensity and duration of individual attacks.

All our knowledge used in relieving muscular and vascular head pain seems useless in fighting the last two categories of headaches. Trigeminal neuralgia, the most severe pain of all, seems unaffected by relaxation therapy or drug therapy, or even by severing the nerve that causes the pain. And of course, headache caused by disease can be relieved only when the disease is treated.

Let's look at these four categories of head pain and see how they can affect you.

Muscle-Contraction Headaches

I like to use the term muscle-contraction headache rather than tension headache because pain caused by tight, spastic muscles doesn't occur only in emotionally tense situations. Tight muscles can result from poor posture, from working in awkward positions, and from a too sudden strain. Stress, however, does remain the most common catalyst that transforms a painless muscle-tension condition into a chronic ache.

The stress can be emotional: You can have a fight with your spouse or boss and boil inside for hours. Or it can be environmental: If a new building is being constructed in your backyard, the unusual noise can keep you on edge. Whatever the stimulus is, the body will react the same way to all stress. All your muscles will be tensed up, ready to fight or flee. Since you don't take any action, the tension continues to build until the muscles become sore and cause pain.

While we all must endure the environmental stresses of our competitive society, not everyone suffers chronic headaches. Why do some people collapse under the same pressure that others seem to thrive on? We used to think that the only reason was some inherent trait that made one person more susceptible to stress than another. Each of us has a different stress threshold, which allows one person to cope easily with misfortune, major life events and success while another suffers fits of anxiety in the face of a minor crisis. The anxious individual is more prone to headaches than is the less affected person.

Temperament is often a factor in muscle-contraction headaches, but we've found that many people also have skeletal imbalances ch make them more susceptible to stress-induced pain. We scussed the most common imbalance affecting headaches in the previous chapter—the jaw imbalance. Because the head, shoulder and neck muscles are straining already to compensate for the unbalanced jaw structure, they are easy targets for the muscle tension produced by an argument, an exam, a sudden loud noise or an important event. Little stress other than the jaw imbalance is needed to cause muscle spasms and pain.

Muscle-contraction headaches present a rather ironic situation. They are at once the most frequently suffered long-term pain in this country, and the easiest of the head pains to treat. The key to relieving the pain is in discovering the cause of the muscle tension. It is in this area that most diagnosticians fall short. They are uneducated in the role of the TMJ Syndrome, or jaw imbalance, in causing headaches.

Without this information about muscular headaches, many practitioners will treat a "tension" headache with tranquilizers and painkillers. The object of such regimens is to relieve anxiety and relax the muscles pharmacologically. There may be relief after these medications are used for a month or six weeks, but the effects of the drugs will wear off. The sufferer will need more and more medication to shake a headache. And since the drugs only serve to cover up the tension, they won't get to the root of the muscle-contraction pain. They can't help reposition an imbalanced jaw, nor can they teach you to control the pent-up tension in your muscles.

My message comes down to this: If you suffer from chronic muscle-contraction headaches, you can't find relief in a bottle of pills. Getting through the day on painkillers and tranquilizers is not conquering the pain. You're just ignoring a message that your body is sending—a distress signal. The longer you ignore that message, the more pills you'll have to take to quiet it.

Work with your body. If you have muscle-tension pain, find out where the tension is coming from. Your posture could be the culprit. Make mental notes about how you hold your body during the day. For instance, one common cause for headache among office workers is cupping the phone between the shoulder and chin while writing, reaching for some papers or otherwise using the hand that should be holding the phone. If you're on the phone a lot, the muscles in your shoulder, neck and head are going to contract and go into spasm. Soon they'll become painful and you have a headache even though you're feeling calm and relaxed.

Students can develop headaches from hunching over their desks all day with their shoulders tensed up and their heads bent over. The neck and shoulder muscles may be tensed for hours, until they cramp up and cause that familiar dull ache at the nape of the neck and surrounding the head.

If you find that you have posture habits that cause the head, neck and shoulder muscles to remain tensed for long periods of time, make an effort to find better positions for whatever jobs you do.

Maybe it's not the way you hold your body that causes tension. You might find that you tense up under pressure. One quick check for this is to see if your hands are clenched in fists while you're walking or in conversation. This is a signal that your whole body is braced. Try a self-relaxation exercise program like biofeedback or autohypnosis. This will help build up your stress threshold. We've devoted a whole chapter in this book to relaxation programs. You'll find that most require only a few minutes of attention a day, and the exercises can be done at home, in an office, or even while you're riding home from work at night.

Another good method of releasing tension from your body is to take up a sport. It needn't be a competitive one. As a matter of fact, some people find that competition makes them more tense. Solitary exercise like jogging or swimming is an excellent method of keeping your muscles toned and relaxed.

At work, you can use one simple exercise to help keep your neck and shoulder muscles limber. Whenever you feel tension around your head, sit back for a moment and do a few slow head rolls. Bring your chin down to your chest, slowly circle your head to the left, drop it back, bring it to the right and back to your chest. You can do five in one direction, then switch and do five in the other.

Head rolls stretch the muscles you tend to tense under pressure, so that muscle spasms, and the headaches that go with them, can be prevented.

Another step in preventing and controlling muscle-contraction headaches is to keep a headache diary. We've provided a sample page for you here. You can make your own diary in any convenient notebook. Just make sure that you include the following information: Day, time of onset, foods eaten in the last twenty-four hours, emotional climate at time of onset, activity at time of onset, unusual life events occurring close to onset, duration of headache, what relieved it.

Since seven or eight out of ten muscle-contraction-headache sufferers have a jaw imbalance, give yourself the tests presented in Chapter 2 to see if you can identify an unbalanced jaw. If you have any of the symptoms connected with the TMJ Syndrome, see a specialist for a confirmed diagnosis and the proper treatment.

Finally, you should be aware of the danger signals for headache sufferers. You may think that a headache that has lasted for seven years must indicate some life-threatening disease. Just the opposite is true. The longer you have a familiar kind of headache, the more benign it is. Here's what to watch for*:

1. Any severe headache that starts suddenly.
2. Any headache that is accompanied by convulsions.
3. Headache accompanied by fever.
4. Headache accompanied by mental confusion or any drop in conscious awareness or alertness.
5. Headache along with localized pain in an eye or ear or any specific area.
6. Headache following a blow on the head.
7. Headaches starting suddenly in old people.
8. Recurring headaches in children.
9. Any headache that interferes with daily living.

*Reprinted from *Headaches: The Kinds and the Cures,* pages 16–18 with permission of author Arthur S. Freese, D.D.S. and publisher, Doubleday & Co., Inc.

DAY	ONSET TIME	WHAT I ATE IN THE LAST 24 HOURS	HOW I FELT WHEN I DEVELOPED THE HEADACHE	WHAT I WAS DOING WHEN IT STARTED	UNUSUAL STRESSES	HOW LONG IT LASTED	WHAT MADE THE PAIN STOP
Monday							
Tuesday							
Wednesday							
Thursday							
Friday							
Saturday							
Sunday							

10. Initial occurrence of daily or frequent headaches.
11. A sudden change in the kind of headache you experience.
12. A headache aggravated by coughing, straining or stooping.
13. An unfamiliar headache that awakens you at night. Again, the great majority of headaches are benign. They may make your life miserable, but they won't endanger it.

As you can see from the information here, the proper diagnosis and some attention to personal habits can result in the relief of your head pain without using habituating drugs. The victims of vascular headaches aren't so lucky, as we'll see in the next section.

Vascular Headaches

These are the "sick" headaches. Unlike the dull ache of muscle-contraction headaches, these send throbbing pain into one or both sides of the head during an attack. Vascular headaches are so called because they appear to begin with an inflammation of the blood-vessel walls. According to the most popular theory today, the blood vessel, most often an artery, first constricts; then the blood flow forces it open. This dilation irritates the vessel walls, causing them to become inflamed and painful. When blood passes through to the brain, you feel the throbbing pain that is so characteristic of this family of headaches.

The most common form of this headache is the migraine. A small percentage of migraine sufferers have "classic" migraine, complete with pre-headache aura, which occurs about twenty minutes before the pain starts, causing the victim to lose partial or total vision, experience numbness in the extremities, see lights, hallucinate, have trouble writing and talking, or even pass out. Many researchers believe that this aura occurs when a blood vessel constricts and causes a loss of blood to the brain.

Most migraineurs suffer the common form, however, in which simple light and sound sensitivity precedes the attack.

In either case, the pain grows gradually from an ache to a rhythmic throb on one side of the head. Usually there's some indigestion. Many people can't take their migraine preparation orally because they're so nauseous. Yet without the medication, the attacks are often more intense and prolonged.

In the throes of an attack, a migraine victim can do little but lie in the dark and hope for relief. Attacks average six to eight hours for most people, though they can last for days or weeks. When the pain finally begins to subside, the migraineur usually falls asleep. Upon waking, the pain will be gone, but a washed-out, listless feeling will remain for the rest of the day.

Studies of migraine sufferers have shown us some patterns in the development of these headaches, though little of this information can help in curing the blight. We know that the predisposition for migraines can be passed on genetically. If both your parents have migraines, you stand a 75 percent chance of developing them yourself.

Nine out of ten migraineurs are women. They usually have the first attack either when the menstrual cycle begins or in their early twenties, when adult pressures increase. The episodic headaches continue for about twenty years, usually subsiding after menopause. Often there will be a respite during pregnancy. And for "lucky" women sufferers, the headaches are at least predictable, occurring once a month like clockwork when their menstrual periods are regular. Most migraine attacks, however, have no biological timing. They happen for many reasons, usually at inopportune moments.

Everyone seems to have his or her own idiosyncratic headache pattern. But the precipitators of the individual headaches may be common to all migraines. Researchers have isolated three of the most frequent triggers: ingestion of certain foods, stress, and change in hormone levels.

For those whose headaches are triggered by the abrupt increase or decrease in stress, biofeedback and other exercises used to control the response to stress are prescribed. These people might be suffering from a combination muscle-contraction headache and migraine condition; the tension headache triggers the migraine. We know that any stress—whether it's an upsurge in pressure or the sudden lack of it—can precipitate a muscle-contraction headache.

And as we already discussed, relaxation exercises can increase the stress threshold, thereby relieving the headaches. In patients whose migraines are precipitated by tension headaches, then, relieving the muscular headache can reduce the number of migraine attacks as well.

Though controversy over the role of certain foods in inducing migraine headaches still exists, some specialists in the field swear by their nitrite/alcohol/monosodium glutamate/tyramine-free diet as a standard part of their treatment. All these agents are vasoactive substances: they can cause the blood vessels to dilate or constrict, thereby initiating the migraine process.

Tyramine is found in certain foods, such as aged cheeses, chicken livers, chocolate and red wine. Chinese cuisine is often laced with monosodium glutamate to enhance flavors. The addition of this chemical to almost all Chinese food in restaurants has given rise to the Chinese Restaurant Syndrome. Non-migraineurs suffering from this syndrome develop migrainelike headaches after eating at a Chinese restaurant because of their sensitivity to monosodium glutamate. Nitrite is often found as a preservative in cured meats and lunch meats. If you have vascular headaches, steer clear of bacon, sausage, hot dogs, ham, lunch loaves and salami, as well as any other packaged meats that indicate this ingredient on their wrappers. Finally, there's alcohol. Anyone who has ever had a hangover is familiar with alcohol's vasoactive properties.

We've supplied a list of the foods to take out of your diet if you have vascular headaches. However, to find the individual food triggers that affect you, you should keep a diet chart indicating what you eat every day and when you develop headaches. Some migraineurs aren't affected by foods at all, and this shows up on the diet chart. Along with your diet, you should watch the general pattern of your headaches. Keep a headache diary, like the one described earlier in this chapter for muscle-contraction headaches. The diary will help you recognize other triggers, such as anger or unusual pressure.

Precautionary steps such as increasing the stress threshold and changing a diet can reduce tremendously the number of attacks you suffer. But what can you do about the headaches you do have to live with?

Listed below are seven foods that have the best established reputation as headache producers.*

1. Milk
2. Chocolate
3. Eggs
4. Wheat
5. Peanuts
6. Citrus Fruits (including tomatoes)
7. Pork

Note also that this means that you must analyze the ingredients of the various concoctions that you tend to eat regularly to determine if one of these "big seven" is hidden in your favorite snack and also causing your chronic headaches.

Additionally, food high in tyramine, a food chemical that dilates blood vessels, may be headache inducers. The list of tyramine-high foods includes the following:*

Dairy Products: Aged cheeses, yogurt, sour cream

Meats and Fish: Pickled Herring, salted dried fish, sausages, beef, and chicken livers.

Vegetables: Italian broad beans with pods (fava beans), sauerkraut

Alcoholic Beverages: Beer, ale, red wines, Riesling, sauterne, champagne, sherry

Other: Vanilla, chocolate, yeast and yeast extract, soy sauce

In the last two decades, nearly every large medical center has developed a headache clinic to answer that question. And of course, various points of view have come out of that research. If you have infrequent attacks, many specialists will suggest a cup or two of strong black coffee (caffeine constricts blood vessels) as a preven-

---

*Reprinted from *The Woman's Holistic Headache Relief Book*, pages 42 and 64, with permission of the authors June Bierman & Barbara Toohey and St. Martin's Press.

tive step when you feel an attack coming on. Then get yourself to a
quiet dark room with someone on hand to comfort you. Ride it out
with aspirin, TLC and an ice pack.

Others suggest the use of ergot preparations. These are abortive
medications that catch the headache before it blossoms. For these
medications to be effective, however, you must have some pre-
headache signal. Ergot preparations essentially constrict the blood
vessels before they are fully dilated and inflamed. Once the vessels
are painful, the drug has little effect.

There are drawbacks to this medication. As mentioned earlier in
this chapter, a common side effect is nausea, which, when coupled
with the indigestion accompanying a migraine, may make it
impossible to hold down the drug. The suppository form of ergot
preparations is easier to accept into the system, but less convenient
to take.

Secondly, you can take only a limited amount of these drugs
before they start to create headaches in a rebound effect. People who
suffer frequent migraines often abuse their prescriptions and, after a
few weeks, develop a continuous headache until the drug is flushed
out of their system.

Migraineurs whose attacks occur three or four times a week have
few treatment alternatives. Most specialists suggest a combination
of drugs for these sufferers. One of the most effective medications is
Sansert, but it is also one of the most dangerous drugs. You can only
take this for a few months at a time, break for six weeks and then
continue treatment. Even under these conditions, prolonged use is
not recommended.

Researchers in the field have looked into antidepressants and
some hypertension medications as safe alternatives to Sansert and
ergot preparations. For some reason yet unknown, antidepressant
drugs, such as Elavil, and blood-pressure preparations seem to be
successful in controlling many migraine problems. Although these
drugs also have side effects, which must be considered before taking
them for long periods, they offer fewer hazards than other migraine
pharmacotherapies. And for many headache sufferers, minor side

effects are often a blessing if the drug with which they are associated can promise relief.

I'd like to point out here that frequent migraine attacks necessitating this kind of drug therapy are unusual. Migraines occurring three and four times a week often indicate a combination headache problem. You may actually suffer three or four muscle-contraction headaches a week, which are triggering the vascular head pain. In these cases, as we discussed earlier, controlling the muscular headaches would lessen the frequency of the vascular attacks.

Another confusing factor in distinguishing true migraines from frequent severe headaches is the trigger point. This muscular problem can mimic migraine pain. The trigger point that forms in a left-shoulder muscle spasm, for example, can refer pain to the left side of the head—a throbbing, stabbing pain that can be continuous. Misdiagnosis of this muscular problem as a migraine condition happens frequently. Of course, any migraine preparation used to treat this headache wouldn't relieve it. You'd have to treat the source of the muscle tension to stop the pain.

It makes sense, then, to be checked for tension headaches even though your head pain appears to be strictly vascular. Use your headache diary to look for a pattern showing an increase in migraines when you're under tension. You can try biofeedback and other relaxation techniques as a means of relieving tension head pain.

Also, look for signs that your posture is causing the muscles to cramp up and cause pain. These muscle spasms can be relieved only by changing your work position, or your reading posture, or the chair in which you watch TV, for example. If you hold your body in such a way that all the parts are supported properly, the muscles will be able to relax.

Above all, you can test yourself for the TMJ Syndrome. Since a jaw imbalance is behind 75 percent of all muscle-contraction headaches, it only makes sense to be examined for this disorder. Many of our patients have come in with continual devastating migraines that actually were triggered by the TMJ Syndrome. When their jaws were balanced and the muscles in the head and neck treated, the migraines subsided in frequency and intensity to where they were no longer a problem. I'll let just one of them tell you for herself:

Paula

"My family has a history of migraines, so when I started to get severe headaches at sixteen, everyone shook their head and said, 'Poor kid, she's got them too. Maybe she'll grow out of them.' I didn't. I grew into them. When I was in college, I'd have two or three killers a week. I'd just sit in the phone booth in my dormitory and wail long distance to my parents.

"I had already seen a neurologist before I went to college and was assured that my brain was functioning perfectly. So at school, I visited a general practitioner. He gave me some migraine medication and said that I'd have to learn to live with the attacks. 'Under stress, some people cry,' he said, shrugging, 'some get stomach aches, and you get headaches.' He also suggested that I see a psychotherapist in an effort to calm down.

"Just as I was about to leave school and live on my own, then, I started seeing a therapist. I had also managed to get a large, refillable prescription for codeine, which I took liberally to keep up with classes. In an effort to clear up these increasingly debilitating headaches before I went out on my own, my father called some twenty-six neurologists and special clinics to get help. One said that for a year and twenty thousand dollars he could cure me. Another suggested a short stay at an institution. Most, however, said to stick with the medication and make the most of my pain-free time.

"Once I settled into my new home and job, the amount of pain-free time I had diminished rapidly. I resolved to visit a headache clinic in the area. After the countless blood tests, medical examinations and x-rays, the specialists gave me the same advice as the doctor at school, with a prescription for a stronger painkiller. Within six weeks, the drug lost its effectiveness when taken as directed.

"I visited another clinic and was given new combination drug treatments, none of which were very safe, but a few of which seemed to ease the pain. I had been working about six months at that time. The headaches were attacking every night more severely than the last. Sometimes I'd have two in one day. Sometimes I'd be sort of paralyzed from the pain, waiting on a corner for my husband to pick me up and lead me home. Other times, I'd just rip at my hair, trying to make the throbbing stop at night so I could go to sleep.

"Finally, my neurologist hit on a combination of drugs that worked, but that I could only take for six months at a time. I gained fifty pounds from one of the drugs. I was fat, but fat doesn't hurt. However, that same drug made me depressed and, eventually, suicidal. When it was discontinued, the headaches started again with a vengeance. I quit work.

"To avoid bankruptcy, I tried to do some free-lance work. On one of these assignments, for a dental magazine, I visited a specialist in TMJ disorders. He just looked at me and said, 'I'll bet you have headaches, and I can cure them.' Well, I don't like medical hocus-pocus, but I was at wits' end. He also mentioned that his program didn't involve drugs or surgery. I was beyond hope or trust, so I certainly had nothing to risk. The next day, I started being treated for a jaw imbalance.

"Whenever I say what I'm going to say next, people always say, 'Oh, come on.' But it's true. In two months, after I had the acrylic appliance put in my mouth, I was pain-free and off all medications. In five months, I dropped all the weight I'd put on because of the drug therapy. I was, essentially, cured.

"The real test of this cure came four months after I'd had my last headache. I broke my leg and was on crutches and the migraines came back. No sooner had I written off that treatment than the TMJ specialist explained how I'd knocked off the balance again while on crutches. He adjusted the bite plate, and the headaches, as abruptly as they had reappeared, vanished."

Many people with migraine headache feel as if their brains are somehow causing the pain or at least being injured by these terrible attacks. The intensity of most vascular headaches would certainly give the sufferer reason to believe that this is so. But, as with muscular headaches, the severity of the pain often is not an indicator of the danger it presents. Many long sufferers of migraines have retained their wit and intelligence. To date, no brain damage has been known to result from severe migraine attacks. However, you should watch for certain danger signals in migraine, as well as those given earlier in this chapter for all headaches, that could suggest a serious disease:*

1. Medication that usually works becoming suddenly useless
2. Any changes in personality or mental functions
3. A headache that dramatically turns sudden and severe
4. Physical or neurological changes (sight, speech, feeling or paralysis, for example) that last after the headache is gone
5. Signs of any sort of disease

   If you recognize any of these signs, see your physician immediately.

Cluster: the man's migraine

   Cluster headaches are vascular, like migraines. But that is where the similarity ends. Ninety percent of the time, cluster strikes men between forty and sixty years of age. The attacks are tightly bunched together in "clusters." They occur without warning, cruelly waking the victim out of a sound sleep. The burning, boring pain starts abruptly on one side of the face in the eye and temple and lasts from twenty to ninety minutes. Often the painful eye becomes bloodshot and teary, and the nostril on that side becomes stuffy and runs. Otherwise mature and sedate men have been known to dance wildly around their office during attacks, holding the painful side of their head. Some try to smash the pain out against a wall, and others tear at their hair in an attempt to rip the pain out.

---

*Reprinted from *Headaches: The Kinds and the Cures,* 1973, page 49, with permission from author Arthur S. Freese, D.D.S. and publisher, Doubleday & Co., Inc.

A cluster sufferer can have a dozen or more of these attacks in a day. Sometimes the headaches will stretch over a week or longer. Then, as mysteriously as they appeared, the attacks will disappear for a few months or even several years.

As in the cases of other vascular headaches, researchers have found no specific pattern in or cause for cluster attacks. We know that some men are particularly prone to these headaches during the fall and spring. Others seem to develop headaches whenever a change in the emotional climate occurs. Still other headaches seem related somehow to a chemical present in the body tissue itself—histamine. Histamine is a vasodilator which can kick off this vascular headache when its level rises in the bloodstream.

The role of vasoactive agents aside from histamine is perplexing. All the chemicals that affect migraineurs, like alcohol, tyramine, nitrites and monosodium glutamate, can also trigger a cluster attack, but only when the sufferer is predisposed to the headaches. During the months or years when the headaches are in remission, the cluster victim can eat or drink anything without worry. However, the unpredictable nature of these headaches makes it impossible to know the safe periods.

Preventive action for cluster attacks is difficult to take. The headaches are so sudden that migraine preparations, which can be effective on all vascular headaches, can't be taken early enough to abort the headache. At the same time, long-term medication seems inappropriate for a head pain that may occur only for one week in three months. So infrequent cluster headache sufferers can rely on little other than strong painkillers to lessen the intensity of the pain they endure.

Persistent cluster headaches striking two and three times a week, however, require some kind of prevention program. Often the ergot preparations used in ongoing migraine problems can be effective in halting attacks. But even preparations that are developed to be used every day can usually be prescribed for only six months at a time. After six months, then, you're back to square one.

One tactic used in some headache clinics is desensitization. Specialists inject the headache sufferer with histamine just below the critical level that would trigger an attack. Over a period of time, you're supposed to become less susceptible to histamine as a triggering agent. However, histamine's role in cluster headaches is still ill defined. Therefore, this treatment remains of speculative value.

Another approach to prevention is to identify the specific triggers of an individual's headaches. This is best done by consulting a headache diary compiled by the sufferer over several months. Any foods that seem to play a role in the attacks are taken out of the diet forever. And if stress plays a prominent part, relaxation training will be employed to keep tension at a minimum. With perseverance and a little luck, you can avoid many cluster episodes and lessen the intensity of those you do suffer through by using the right combination of medication and relaxation techniques.

Like migraineurs, cluster-headache victims feel that the pain they endure must be doing some irreparable damage to their mental abilities. It isn't. However, you should be on the watch for the same warning signals that apply to migraine victims.

Cluster and migraine headaches are indeed hard to live with. It's difficult to imagine a chronic headache that causes more agony than a vascular one. However, the facial neuralgias present a head pain so severe that people consider taking their life rather than live through another attack.

Facial Neuralgia

Tic douloureux, or trigeminal neuralgia, is the most common of the facial neuralgias. It strikes suddenly, with full force, lancing one side of the face with a devastating pain. Like clusters, you might have five attacks in one week, then be untroubled for a year or more. The tic's course is completely unpredictable.

We're not sure what starts this horrible head pain, nor what can stop it. We do know, however, where the pain comes from—the trigeminal nerve. This nerve provides feeling for your jaws and face—for the nose, lips, cheeks, mouth, tongue, eyes, teeth and gums. You have two, one for each side of the head. To our best understanding, the trigeminal nerve is aggravated by a trigger action, like eating, breathing, blowing the nose, laughing, swallowing or yawning, or by the slightest pressure on a trigger area such as the lips, nose, cheeks or forehead.

Ordinarily, tic sufferers face a brisk wind or sip a drink like the rest of us. But on occasion, without warning, such triggers as these will cause an explosion of searing pain on one side of the face. The first spasm may last for twenty or thirty seconds. Then, just as you begin to feel safe for a few seconds, another attack will grab the side of your face. These spasms may continue for an hour or more, each striking more severely than the previous one.

The pain of tic douloureux is so intense that once trigger areas and actions are isolated, victims will avoid them at all costs. If the trigger is on a man's cheek, he may grow a beard so that he doesn't have to shave that one spot. A woman with the same trigger might avoid washing that area or applying make-up to it. Someone with a chewing trigger will live on a liquid diet; a person with a swallowing trigger won't let food or water pass his or her lips for fear of encouraging this terrible pain.

Tic douloureux strikes middle-aged or older people—usually women. Researchers do have a theory about the cause of this pain, although it is not yet proved: The trigeminal nerve in a healthy body is separated by a bone from the major artery running near it. In people suffering trigeminal neuralgia, however, that bone may be defective or somehow degenerated so that only a thin layer of tissue separates the nerve from the artery. In postmenopausal women, demineralization of the bone would allow the nerve to lie too close to the artery. The artery would then aggravate the nerve when one of the trigger mechanisms was activated. The pulsations of the artery would account for the throbbing nature of the tic's pain.

What kind of help is available for the person suffering with this unpredictable, devastating tic? Specialists who treat the disease have tried a combination of therapies designed to cope with this condition, which becomes increasingly severe and more resistant to treatment with each attack.

Usually the therapy will start off with drugs. One in use now is Dilantin. This may help as a preventive measure for a short time. Then stronger medication will be called for. When the drugs lose their effectiveness, treatment is aimed at numbing the nerve itself. It may be injected with alcohol to produce long-term anesthesia. Sometimes hot water is injected into the nerve, providing a shock that seems to stall any tic episodes for a few months. Each injection of alcohol or hot water, however, will last a shorter time than the previous treatment. Soon another, more drastic approach is necessary.

The next step is to sever the nerve. The first time this surgery is performed, relief may last for as long as a year and a half. Then the severing will have to be performed again, the nerve cut off closer to the brain. This time the respite will be shorter, and another operation required in another six months. Finally, even this procedure will lose its effectiveness.

Another attempt to destroy the nerve and stop the tic permanently involves running a radio-frequency current through the nerve via a conductor needle. This is a promising technique—simple and safe. However, we are still unsure of the duration of the relief that even this procedure can ensure.

One operation used today focuses not on destroying the nerve, but on moving it away from the artery so that the pulsing vessel won't press on it and create the terrific pain spasms. Some sufferers have found that this procedure has cured the tic. But since we know of no absolute cause of trigeminal neuralgia, we can only promise that this surgery will be successful for those people whose tics are caused by the proximity of an artery to the trigeminal nerve.

It has also been found, however, that the TMJ Syndrome may be a factor in tic douloureux. We have had cases where the painful episodes subsided when the jaw balance was reestablished. Other times, the repositioning of the jaw was combined with destroying the nerve in a tooth that was singled out as a trigger by the sufferer. This procedure has been especially successful in those sufferers who can recognize exactly which teeth are trigger areas.

Treatment of tic douloureux with a TMJ Syndrome regimen is by no means 100 percent effective. However, we believe that this procedure should be included in the diverse methods used to combat this pain, since it can be successful in certain cases.

Finally, an answer for the tic's pain that doesn't include drugs or surgery is the transcutaneous nerve stimulator, introduced by Dr. C. Norman Shealy, a neurologist and a leader in the battle against pain. Dr. Shealy's device sends an electric current into the nerve that is transmitting the pain signal. The current apparently scrambles the pain message to the brain, thereby eliminating the discomfort. Though this device is relatively new, the electronic stimulator has performed well in many of the cases for which it was prescribed, including chronic backache, neckache and headache. It has helped people with virtually uncontrollable pain, like tic douloureux, to return to normal life styles.

Like vascular headaches, trigeminal neuralgia may make mature men and women stamp around a room and tear their hair as a result of the pain, but the attacks are harmless. Once the episode is over, no permanent damage is evident. Ironically, headaches caused by tumors or other deadly diseases seem minor next to the horrendous pain of a vascular or tic douloureux head pain—at least in their initial stages.

Traction (a pulling or stretching by the extension of a growth or inflammatory process) and Inflammatory Headaches: Quiet and Deadly

A thirty-four-year-old newlywed and his bride are driving across the country. They're honeymooning in Arizona. Bob develops a persistent dull ache in his head. He figures it's from watching the road too long. After two days, the eye behind which most of the pain is concentrated starts to water and becomes bloodshot. It must be some allergy or other, he thinks.

In Arizona, Bob and his wife visit an ear-nose-and-throat specialist. "It looks like you have a little infection," the doctor says, "but to make sure, let's take an x-ray."

The next day, Bob goes back for the results and the doctor seems strangely apprehensive. "We didn't find anything wrong with your sinuses," he says, "but we did find the cause of your headaches."

Bob had a brain tumor the size of a baseball in his head, yet he suffered only mildly annoying headaches.

How can this be possible? How can slight irritation to a nerve or irregular blood flow in an artery cause unbearable pain while a tumor the size of a fist causes a two-aspirin headache? The answer lies in the brain itself. It doesn't feel pain. You can drill into it, poke at it or cut into it and you won't feel a thing. So when a brain tumor develops, it won't become noticeable in the form of a headache until it's large enough to cause the brain tissues to pull and press on sensitive tissues in the head—the blood vessels and nerves lying around the brain itself.

Of course, headache isn't the only symptom of a brain tumor or of other dangerous diseases whose symptoms include head pain. You could feel suddenly dizzy or have other neurological signs, like loss of balance, numbness and weakness in some part of the body, or loss of one of your senses. These are some of the danger signals that we listed earlier in this chapter. Again, if any of these signs appear, see your physician immediately.

What the Four Categories Mean to You

Of the 42 million Americans suffering headaches, approximately ninety percent have muscle-contraction pain, 8 percent are afflicted with vascular headaches, and only 2 percent have traction and inflammatory conditions.

This percentage breakdown has its good and bad points. Obviously, it means that most of you with headaches that have been plaguing you for seven years have nothing to worry about. Your head pain is just that—an ache in the head, which doesn't indicate any serious threat to your health.

The bad part, of course, is that chronic pain makes life miserable—whether it's caused by muscle contraction or by disease. And the treatments you may try to get rid of that persistent noxious pain can have deleterious effects on your health. Drugs, perhaps the most common therapy for headaches, can make you nauseous, depressed, anxious, restless, dizzy, drowsy. Just read the label: it's written in black and white for you.

We're not saying that all drugs are bad. They can work miracles for many kinds of illness. But they can't cure pain. They just cover it up. For most chronic headache victims, we offer an alternative, often permanent relief of pain.

Only one other pain besides headache affects as many people, and that is the backache—the subject of our next chapter.

Aching Backs: What Causes Them?

"I don't understand it," he says. "I just bent down to pick up a dime—*a dime*—and my back went out. I couldn't move for four days." Sound familiar to you? How many times have you shoveled snow, raked leaves or changed a tire, only to find that after you were finished, you couldn't straighten out your back for a day. This is just a taste of what a chronic sufferer lives with every day. Backache victims aren't a medical elite, either. They are second in number only to headache sufferers. American doctors see patients with back pain 18,824,000 times a year.

With all this practice, you'd think that physicians could cure a pain in the back with their hands tied. Unfortunately, that's far from the case. Many of those 18,824,000 office visits are from repeaters, people who have tried one method of pain control that failed and have come back for another. Are our backs that poorly constructed that picking up a dime, or carrying out the garbage, or bending over an ironing board, inevitably will cause chronic pain?

Some specialists feel that indeed a major cause of back disorders is the fact that we're orthopedic lemons. Our nine-to-fourteen pound heads rest uneasily on our broomstick-figure skeletal frames. Most of us don't kneel down to pick up heavy loads; we bend over and hoist them up. We don't use our arms and legs to help out the back. We just pull it, twist it, hunch it, weigh it down, and then expect the muscles surrounding that weak link of vertebrae to endure for a lifetime under this abuse.

True, some of our carrying and posture habits are detrimental to our back, but that's not the main problem. We could handle many more twists, sudden movements and heavy weights if our back muscles—the real workhorses—weren't knotted up from too little exercise and excessive stress. Eighty percent of the backaches in this country are caused by stress and muscle strain.

Backache is a disease of civilization—an offshoot of our energy-saving, time-conserving technology, which reduces most physical labor to mere button pushing. Many of our jobs are desk-oriented, sedentary positions. Getting up and going to work along with coming home and eating dinner can take up your day from seven in the morning to seven at night. So who has time to exercise, right? The longer you sit without stretching those back muscles, be it in the office or in front of the TV at home, the less elastic and weaker your back becomes.

Stress and Backache

Compounding this sedentary abuse is stress. The stress syndrome described in Chapter 2 applies to the back as well as anywhere else in the body. When you're under pressure, or the boss decidedly dislikes you last piece of work, or there's a new buzzer used on the intercom in your office which you find particularly annoying, or you're subjected to any of the innumerable irritants of everyday life, your body is getting ready either to flee from the distress or to combat it. Adrenaline is pumped into the system. You're ready for action, but you don't do anything. You just sit at your desk or stand at the sink or continue to do whatever it was that you were supposed to be doing. What happens to all that tension in the muscles? It stays there.

If your back muscles are stiff from lack of exercise, they're the perfect repository for this kind of stress-induced tension. Every day, those back muscles tense up a little more, become a little less elastic, and are unable to expand to their full resting position. Then one day, you move the wrong way while changing a light bulb or picking up a pencil, and your back muscles go into acute spasm, causing great pain and immobility.

Some of us have been made sufficiently aware of the detrimental effects of our inactive life styles to cause us to do something about our physical conditions. However, there are good and bad ways to become physically fit. Let's look at one fellow who decided after many years to tune his body into the fine instrument that it had been during college.

Mr. J. is a successful professional. He works hard at his desk, crouched over papers, the phone hooked to his ear with his shoulder. Lunching with clients often means a few drinks and veal parmigiana for lunch. After work, he likes to go to movies, the theater or sports events with his family. And on weekends, he manages to get in a few hours on the golf course. Even with all this activity, Mr. J. noticed that his paunch was taking up more and more space between the desk and his chair.

One day he decided to get into an exercise regimen, a little jogging before he went to work. Mr. J. bought himself a new runner's suit and a pair of Pumas. The next day he rolled out of bed, into his new shoes and out onto the pavement. A half hour later, winded, he decided not to overdo and walked briskly back home. He took a shower and sat down to breakfast with the paper.

In a perfectly ordinary manner, Mr. J. leaned over to get the milk, and it happened. His back locked painfully in one position. He thought for sure that it was broken. But his problem was muscular. It was the first of many episodes like this that he'd have in his life.

What happened? Wasn't Mr. J. doing the right thing? Aren't we supposed to be getting into shape?

The answer is yes. Exercise is recommended for everyone to keep the muscles toned and to release tension. But this man, like many other people, didn't start exercising by stretching out those tense, tight back muscles. They couldn't absorb the shock of sudden activity, and that trauma caused them to go into spasm. Many first episodes of back pain start when a person decides to do leg lifts or sit-ups after years of inactivity, but fails to begin the exercise period with warm-up stretching.

After his experience vith jogging, Mr. J. decided to take it easy. No lifting, no more crazy strenuous exercises. Work and golf he knew were safe and Mr. J. wasn't taking any more chances with his back.

The decision to return to a completely sedentary life was probably more detrimental to Mr. J.'s back muscles than the original decision to jog. His muscles are already in spasm. Without proper exercise, they'll continue to grow stiffer and weaker. His backache attacks will become more frequent and intense. Soon he may find that there's pain radiating down one of his legs. That's the trigger points starting to develop in the back muscles—those little nodules of degenerated tissue that can send sharp pains shooting into the calf or thigh.

After a few years of tranquilizers, biweekly visits to a back specialist, and disabling pain, Mr. J. finds himself in a hospital getting ready to have a disk removed or a spinal fusion. In reality, nothing is wrong with his spine; the knotted, tense muscles are causing all the pain.

Other Causes of Back Pain

Stress and tension are the two most frequent purveyors of backache, but other factors unrelated to our emotional natures can cause back discomfort too.

Skeletal imbalance, for instance, is a cause of discomfort in some muscular backaches. Any skeletal imbalance in your body will put stress on the muscle tissue from head to toe. In the case of a short leg, your back muscles are going to be pulling and twisting to keep you from looking too lopsided, and to keep you balanced on two uneven legs. That strain alone is enough to make the muscles sore and tired. Add to it stress, overexertion or too little exercise, and you have the perfect setup for chronic back pain.

Pregnancy is a high-ranking cause of chronic back problems. The abdominal wall is weakened during pregnancy, and then further taxed when the mother is constantly picking up and carrying the baby. Rather than make the legs and arms do the stooping, hoisting and carrying, many mothers are apt to throw all the weight on the back without stretching and relaxing the muscles after a heavy work load.

Posture is another key component in back distress. Many of us read or watch TV propped up at angles awkward for our back muscles. It's not hard to tell if your position isn't supportive of the back. When you stand up after an hour or so, see if your back is tight and cramped. If so, your lounging posture is poor. Propping yourself up on pillows in bed to read, for instance, is hard on the back. So is sinking into a cushiony reading chair. You don't have to restrict yourself to severe wooden benches; just look for seating that provides a minimal amount of cushioning for comfort, ample support for the whole back, as well as an attractive design.

Housework is another back tormentor. Homemakers or custodians who spend hours every day crouched over the laundry, the ironing or a sponge mop, who lug around heavy cleaning equipment, and who rarely use their arms and legs to support heavy objects that must be moved, are guaranteed back troubles. One way to avoid some backache episodes and to keep the pain from becoming severe is to make sure that during the daily chores, you take time out to stretch the back muscles. And of course, you should kneel when lifting a laundry basket, and try to stand straight while ironing or cleaning. These posture habits will keep the brunt of the daily strain from falling on the back muscles.

Endocrine imbalances often go unrecognized as a contributor to many muscular pains, including backache. Borderline hypothyroidism and estrogen deficiency, the two most common hormone disorders we see, can result in muscle cramps, weakness and soreness. In our histories, we always include the following questions to help identify these conditions. You may want to write your answers to them:

1. Does your hair fall out?
2. Is your skin dry?
3. Do your nails break easily?
4. Do you need an inordinate amount of sleep?

5. Do you have a weight problem?
6. Are your periods regular?
7. Are you always cold?
8. Do you have a problem with constipation?
9. Do you have difficulty conceiving?
10. How is your period?*

Affirmative answers to these questions could mean that endocrine imbalances are playing a part in your back-pain problem, though lack of exercise and tension are surely accountable too.

These are the most frequent precipitators of muscular back distress. When you attempt to relieve back pain of this kind, you have to attack it simultaneously from all angles. Unfortunately, when we get backaches, most of us will go to bed, try not to stretch or reach for anything, and allow the pain to subside. Then, like Mr. J., we'll try to avoid strenuous activity, fearing that exercise will cause another episode. Yet physical activity is the only means, in many cases, to release the built-up tension in the painful muscles, tone them, and make the back strong and pain-free again.

Muscular vs. "Disk" Pain

Trigger points form as a result of muscle deficiency. When they appear, you can often feel sharp pain radiating down the leg, in the buttocks, or into other areas of the back, along with the constant ache in the back. Many specialists take these shooting pains as fairly accurate indicators of a disk disorder, and prescribe surgery. They may suggest as little motion as possible until an operation is performed. So you stay off your feet as much as you can, letting the tension build up more and more as you worry over the operation. And of course, the symptoms continue or become worse because you're not relaxing the muscles.

Finally, you go in for the surgery. After the allotted time for your recovery, you find that you're no better off, or possibly even worse

*From *Clinical Treatment of Back & Neck Pain*, 1970, pages 21 and 22, with permission of author Hans Kraus, M.D., and publisher, McGraw Hill, Inc.

off, than when you went into the hospital. How could you be better? The muscles, the source of the pain, haven't been treated at all.

We have a number of ways to discern a muscular back pain from a disk disorder. You might use them to understand your own problem better:

1. If you notice a sharp pain radiating from one point in your back when you lie down on a hard surface, you have an indication that a trigger area has developed in your aching back muscles. When you lie down, the trigger points are pressed under the weight and you feel a shooting pain.
2. Pain associated with certain activities usually indicates that you're performing incorrectly somehow. You could be twisting or bending in an awkward manner often enough to pull or irritate muscles.
3. Immediate onset of pain after a movement, a lightning, stabbing kind of pain radiating out from the immediate area of discomfort, often means that the problem is in the spine itself, like a ruptured disk. However, if a period of time elapses between the onset of the pain and the last physical exertion, the discomfort is usually a muscular one.
4. Loss of strength, reflex, sensation and control of bodily functions all reflect a disk rather than a muscular disorder.
5. If you can pinpoint the pain rather exactly, the discomfort is usually due to a trigger point.*

Keep in mind that any neurological loss is cause for concern. If you feel numbness, weakness, pins and needles, or other odd sensations in your legs, something probably is irritating the spinal nerve. Your condition can be quite serious if you lose control of your bowels or urination. For any of these symptoms, the immediate attention of a neurologist or neurosurgeon is required.

---

*From *Clinical Treatment of Back & Neck Pain,* 1970, pages 23 and 24, with permission of author Hans Kraus, M.D., and publisher, McGraw Hill, Inc.

Treating Muscular Back Pain

A few sure indicators of disk problems exist, as we mentioned above. However, the majority of backache complaints fall into a nondescript category, giving most specialists difficulty in assigning a muscular or a spinal origin. Often, after a patient endures years of suffering, the surgeon may suggest an operation in the hope that it will help, even though there may not be proof that the disk to be removed is causing the pain.

We suggest that for most backaches, the safest and most effective method of treatment is this three-step procedure:

1. Check for skeletal imbalance, such as a short leg or an unbalanced jaw.
2. Treat the trigger points.
3. Exercise to restore elasticity and strength to muscles.

You can start this regimen at home. Look in a mirror and check the level of your hips. Are they even? If one is higher than the other, then one of your legs is shorter than the other. Also, do the tests for the TMJ Syndrome described in Chapter 3. If you discover one or both of these imbalances, seek out the help of a specialist to confirm your suspicions and provide the proper treatment. The balancing of the jaw, as described in Chapter 3, is as easy as inserting an acrylic bite plate in the mouth. For a leg or foot disparity, a shoe lift or a form of arch support is often suggested.

These are not difficult procedures, but they can determine the outcome of the rest of your therapy. Any other treatments you try may not be successful without the proper balance of your skeletal system.

Let's say that you are being treated for your leg or jaw imbalance. Your next step would be to have the back specialist find and treat the trigger points in your muscles. When these have been dissolved, you'll notice the absence of the sharp pains that these trigger areas refer down the leg. Your muscles, however, may remain tense and sore for some time after trigger-point therapy (described in Chapter 3).

Hot and cold packs will help the muscles relax more as well as relieve some of the discomfort that you're experiencing. We also find that surface anesthetics are helpful, when used in conjunction with stretching exercises. Ethyl fluoride or Fluori-Methane sprayed periodically over the entire sore area relieves pain and loosens tightness. You hold the bottle ten to twelve inches from the painful area and spray, using even back-and-forth movements, until a white film just begins to form on the skin.

Massage, too, can bring relief from muscle tension and discomfort. You start with a wide surface massage called effleurage. For this, you lay your hands flat on the sore area and move them in circular movements. You can do this lightly or with vigor for a deeper massage. Then begin the kneading massage. Your fingers should be flexed at all times during this procedure. First you grab the muscles between both thumbs and forefingers. Then you knead them with a slow rolling motion, using the heels of your hands, just as you would knead bread dough.

The Kraus-Weber Tests

While the muscles are being treated with massage, trigger-point therapy, and hot or cold packs, you also begin exercising to stretch and tone the tissue. Dr. Hans Kraus, M.D., a pioneer in backache treatment, has developed an exercise system to test as well as treat muscular back pain.*

To start an exercise program, you should know your limitations as well as how to build up strength in those weak areas. The Kraus-Weber tests below are designed to give you that information. Try to take the tests when a friend or relative is present to help you. And of course, if your physician has forbidden this kind of activity, wait until he or she feels that you can take the tests safely.

---

*All exercises reprinted from *Clinical Treatment of Back and Neck Pain*, 1970, with permission of the author, Hans Kraus, M.D., and publisher, McGraw-Hill, Inc.

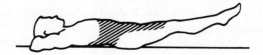

1. Lie flat on your back on the floor with your hands clasped behind your neck, your legs straight and touching. Keeping your knees straight, lift your feet so that your heels are ten inches above the floor, as shown in the above drawing. You pass this test if you can hold that position for ten seconds. This test shows if your hip flexors have sufficient strength.

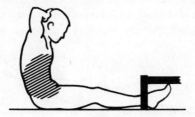

2. Lie flat on the floor again with your hands clasped behind your neck. Have someone hold down your legs by grasping the ankles. If you live alone, hook your ankles under a heavy chair that won't topple. Roll up off the floor, leading with your head, into a sitting position. You pass if you can do one sit-up. This test reveals whether or not your hip flexors and stomach muscles combined are strong enough to handle your body weight.

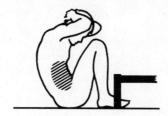

3. Lie flat on the floor with your hands behind your neck and your knees flexed, heels close to the buttocks. Make sure that your

ankles are held down. Then roll up into a sitting position. You pass if you can do one sit-up. This test shows you the strength of your stomach muscles.

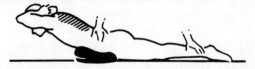

4. Turn over on your stomach. Put a pillow under your abdomen, clasp your hands behind your neck, and lie flat on the floor. Have your helper hold the lower half of your body steady by placing one hand in the small of the back and the other on your ankles. Now lift your trunk and hold it steady for ten seconds. This test reveals whether or not your back muscles are strong.

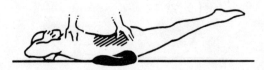

5. Stay on your stomach and clasp your hands behind your neck, making sure that the pillow is still under your abdomen. Have your helper hold your back steady with both hands, as in number 4. Now lift your legs up, keeping your knees straight, and hold the position for ten seconds. This tests the strength of your low-back muscles.

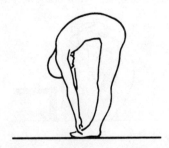

6. Finally, stand up straight and make sure that your feet are together. Relax, lean over, and slowly reach down as far as you can without bending your knees. If you can pass this test, you have sufficient flexibility in your back muscles and hamstrings, the muscles in the back of your thighs. If you fail, it is because these muscles have become shortened and tense, not because your arms are too short or your legs too long.

Corrective Exercises

Now that you know where your weaknesses are, you can begin a program of exercise to strengthen those muscles. The exercises below were developed to provide a tailor-made regimen for every back problem. But even hand-picked exercise courses will not ensure good results. To derive the most from a program, you should keep these points in mind: Once-a-week activity bashes only serve to traumatize the muscles; do your routine every day religiously. Try to perform your exercises in sequence. Built into your routine are the warm-up and cool-down exercises that allow you to work out the muscles without straining them. Finally, never strain the muscles. Feeling a long, painful tug in your back, stomach or anywhere else in your body while exercising doesn't indicate that the muscles are getting stronger. It means that you're pushing too hard.

The first six exercises described here are general muscle-relaxing and limbering movements. You should do all of them, regardless of your problem. These exercises are not endurance tests. We want you to stretch the muscles in one slow continuous movement rather than two quick jerks.

To begin exercising, lie on the floor on a rug or pad. Put pillows under your knees, arms and back for support. Then proceed to go through your exercises, repeating each two or three times in the order they appear and once in reverse. The last exercise you do will be the one with which you began.

1. Loosen up by wobbling your neck, shoulders, arms, thighs, legs and feet. Raise your arms slowly, then let them drop. Repeat these motions with your hands, legs and feet. Let your head drop to the left, then to the right. Take a deep breath—do not strain—exhale slowly.

Now try to feel heavy—let your head, shoulders, arms and legs rest on the floor. Do not attempt to raise yourself by even slightly tensing your muscles.

Breathe deeply again. Close your eyes, let your jaw sag, try to exhale as slowly as possible, humming or hissing.

Tighten your arm muscles, then relax. Tighten your thigh muscles and your neck, then relax. The important part is the relaxing—the letting go—not the tightening. The tightening is important only to make you feel the difference between tension and relaxation.

Breathe deeply again, slowly lift your shoulders to your ears, lower your shoulders, shrug.

2. Get up and shrug your shoulders again.
3. Once more, lie down. Turn your head all the way to the left, then return it to the normal front and center position, and relax. Turn your head all the way to the right, as far as you can, return to normal position, and relax.
4. Lie flat on your back, this time with all pillows removed. Flex your knees and slowly draw your right knee up as close to your chest as possible. Slowly straighten your leg, then let it fall to the floor limp and relaxed. Pull it up again to the flexed starting position. Do the same thing with the other leg. Then repeat the exercise, alternating legs.
5. Lie on your left side, with your head resting comfortably on a pillow and your neck in a relaxed position. Keep both knees flexed and hips slightly flexed. Slide your right knee as close to your head as is comfortably possible, then slowly extend the leg until it is completely straight. Let the leg drop to the floor relaxed. Do the exercise two or three times, then turn to your right side and do the exercise with your left leg.
6. Turn over on your stomach. Let your head rest comfortably on your folded hands. Then tighten your seat muscles. Hold that position for two seconds, then relax.
7. Lie on your back with both knees flexed. Straighten one leg, turn the toes outward, and gradually lift the leg, as illustrated. This exercise is more effective if you add weights when they are

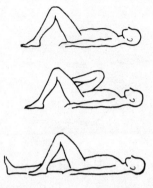

Exercise 4. Flexion-extension while supine

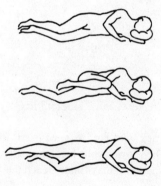

Exercise 5. Flexion-extension while on the side

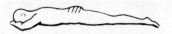

Exercise 6. Gluteal setting

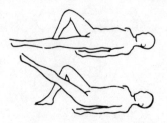

Exercise 7. Rotated leg raise

permitted by your physician. You may use sandbags or light weight-lifting shoes. Start with two pounds, and add only a half pound at a time every second or third day. If you have to jerk or strain, the weight is excessive and should be reduced to the point where you can do it with ease and only slight effort. (This and the next exercise are principally used to strengthen weak hip flexors.)

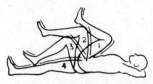

Exercise 8. Heel slide

8. Lie on your back with both knees flexed. Pull both knees up to your chest. Then lower your legs gradually, straightening them at the same time, until they finally reach the floor. Relax.

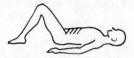

Exercise 9. Abdominal setting

9. Lie on your back with both knees flexed. Tighten your stomach muscles. Try to tighten your seat muscles at the same time. If

you do this correctly, the small of your back will be pressed against the floor. The tight muscles will move your pelvis and bring your back against the floor. You probably will not succeed at once and may have to start by tightening your abdomen and seat muscles separately before you can tighten them together. Once you succeed, hold the muscles tight for two seconds, then relax.

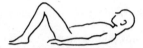

Exercise 10. Head up while supine

10. Lie on the floor, with knees flexed, hands loose by your sides. Raise your head and shoulders off the floor, bring them down slowly and relax. (This and the next two exercises are principally used to strengthen weak stomach or abdominal muscles.)

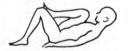

Exercise 11. Knee kiss

11. Lie on your back with knees flexed. Raise your head and your right knee and try to make them meet. Don't try too hard! At first, you will probably not succeed, but eventually you will. Return to your starting position and do the same exercise with your head and left knee.

12. Lie on your back with your hands clasped behind your head, knees flexed. Tuck your feet under a heavy object (a chest of drawers, bed or heavy chair). Be sure that it won't topple over. Sit up, then lower yourself slowly to a lying position. You should sit up gradually, starting by raising your head, then your shoulders, and then your chest and the lower end of the spine. Do not sit up by holding your trunk stiff and jerking your weight

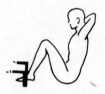

Exercise 12. Sit-up with knees flexed.

up. If you cannot do this exercise with your hands behind your neck, try to do it with your hands at your sides. Later, cross them over your stomach, and still later, when you are stronger, bring your crossed arms up to your chest and finally behind your neck. If you're unable to do this exercise at all, continue with the earlier exercises until you have gained enough strength to manage this one.

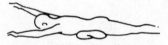

Exercise 13. Single arm raise while prone.

13. Lie on the floor on your stomach with a pillow under your abdomen. Raise your right arm and shoulder, lower them, relax. Do this on alternate sides. (This exercise and the next one are principally used to strengthen upper back muscles.)

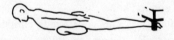

Exercise 14. Back up while prone

14. Lie on your stomach with a large pillow under your waist. Anchor your feet under a heavy piece of furniture that won't topple on you. Keeping your hands at your sides, raise your

back. Raise your back until it is in a horizontal line, but do not arch backward. (Arching-back exercises—so-called hyperextension exercises—may cause discomfort and pain in some patients. Backward arching is not a normal movement of the spine—unless you're an acrobat. Do not do it!)

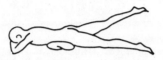

Exercise 15. Single leg raise while prone

15. Lie on your stomach with a large pillow under your waist. Raise one leg, lower it, rest. Raise the other leg, lower it, and rest. (This and the next exercise are used principally to strengthen low-back and seat muscles. However, weakness of the back muscles is rare.)

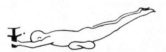

Exercise 16. Double leg raise while prone

16. Lie prone with a pillow under your hips. Anchor your hands by holding on to a solid piece of furniture. Raise both legs together, lower them, rest.
17. The prone stretch. Lie on your stomach, stretch your left arm and right leg as far as you can along the floor, relax. Repeat the exercise with your right arm and left leg. Then stretch with all four limbs at the same time, and relax. (This exercise and the remaining ones are principally used to stretch muscles, from your shoulders to your hamstrings.)
18. Sit on a chair, feet apart on the floor. Let your neck droop, then drop your shoulders and arms, and bend down between your knees, as far as you can. Return to an upright position, straighten up, and relax.

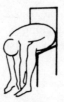

Exercise 18. Bend while sitting

19. Assume a kneeling position, resting on your hands and knees. Arch your back like a cat, and drop your head at the same time. Then reverse the arch by bringing up your head and forming a U with your spine.

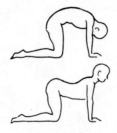

Exercise 19. Cat back

20. Bend sitting rotation. Sit on a chair, bend down, dropping your head and shoulders. Bend down to the left, then gradually straighten up. Rest. Do the exercise again, bending to the right.

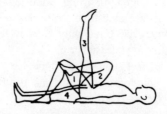

Exercise 21. Hamstring stretch

21. Lie on your back, both knees flexed, arms at your sides. Bring one knee up as close as possible to your face, then raise that leg straight up in the air and lower it slowly to the floor. You should feel a pull in your hamstrings as you do this. Return to the starting position. Relax for a moment before doing the same movement with the other knee.

Exercise 22. Hamstring stretch while standing

22. Stand up, clasp your hands behind your back, keeping your back and neck straight. Bending from the hips, gradually lower your trunk, and go down as far as you can until you feel a stretching of your hamstring muscles.

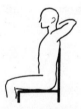

Exercise 23. Pectoral stretch

23. Sit in a chair, place your hands behind your neck, interlace fingers. Now bring your elbows as far back as you possibly can, return to starting position, drop your arms, and relax. Repeat.

24. From a kneeling position, place your hands, then your forearms, on the floor. Gradually straighten your back, sliding forward on your arms and keeping your back and head straight. This will stretch your pectoral muscles as you move away from your knees. Return to a kneeling position, rest, and then repeat the exercise.

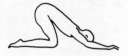

Exercise 24. Kneeling pectoral stretch

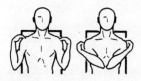

Exercise 25. Upper-back stretch

25. Sit on a chair, your hands placed on your shoulders. Try to cross
your elbows by bringing your right arm as far left as possible
and your left arm as far right as possible until you feel the stretch
across your upper back. Return to starting position, drop your
hands, and relax.

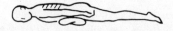

Exercise 26. Shoulder pull while prone

26. Lie on your stomach, a pillow under your hips. Pull your
shoulder blades together, then relax. This exercise can be
helpful in combination with the "shrugging."

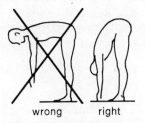

wrong   right

Exercise 27. Floor touch

27. This is the peak exercise given in all programs. To do it, first relax by inhaling and exhaling deeply. Drop your neck gradually and let your trunk "hang" loosely from your hips. Drop your shoulders and then your back gradually. Let gravity help you. Do this two or three times. When you're completely relaxed, "hanging from the hips," reach to the floor as far as you can without straining. Relax again, straighten up, then repeat.

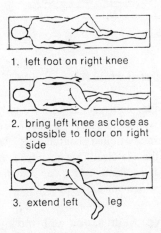

1. left foot on right knee

2. bring left knee as close as possible to floor on right side

3. extend left leg

Exercise 28. Tensor stretch while supine

28. Lie on your back, both legs extended. Bring your left foot up to right knee and rest with the sole of your left foot on your right

knee. Then slowly bring the flexed knee toward the right until
you feel the stretch. Repeat the exercise, alternating sides. This
exercise can be made more effective by extending the knee of
the exercised leg.

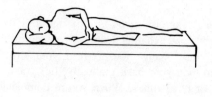

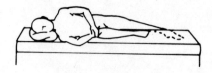

Exercise 29. Tensor stretch while lying on side

29. Lie on your side, with your head on a pillow and both knees
semi-flexed. Extend the upper leg as you bring it as far back as
possible. Return to original position, rest, and turn to your other
side to repeat the exercise. This exercise is best performed on a
hard bed so that the exercised leg can stretch downward, beyond
the surface on which you are lying.

In the following eleven figures, you will find an exercise regimen
designed specifically for your problem as defined by the Kraus-
Weber tests. Remember to repeat each exercise two or three times,
to perform the routine slowly and rhythmically, and to go through
the whole regimen once forward and then once backward.

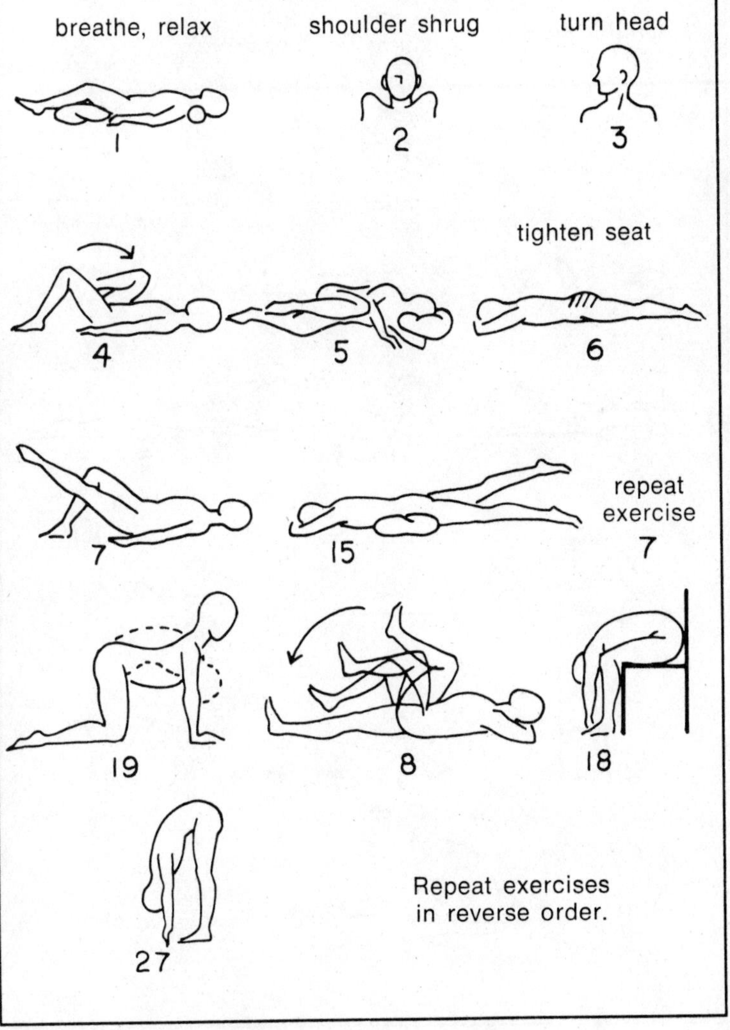

Figure 1: For failure of Kraus-Weber Test 1

Exercises for Weak Hip Flexors and Abdominal Muscles

Do each exercise 2 or 3 times—slowly

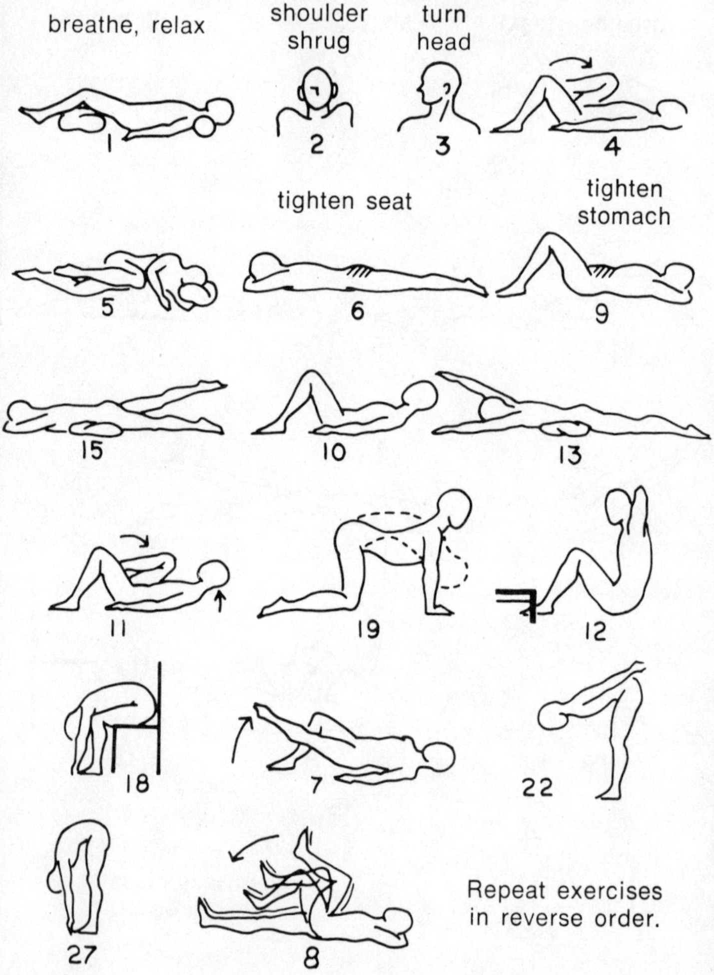

Figure 2: For Failure of Kraus-Weber Test 2

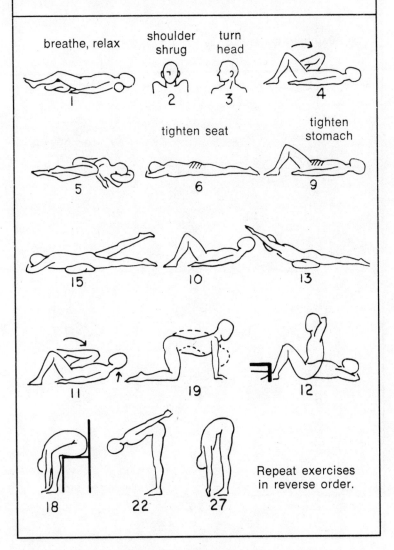

Exercises for Weak Abdominal Muscles

Do each exercise 2 or 3 times—slowly

breathe, relax

shoulder shrug

turn head

1

2

3

4

tighten seat

tighten stomach

5

6

9

15

10

13

11

19

12

18

22

27

Repeat exercises in reverse order.

Figure 3: For Failure of Kraus-Weber Test 3

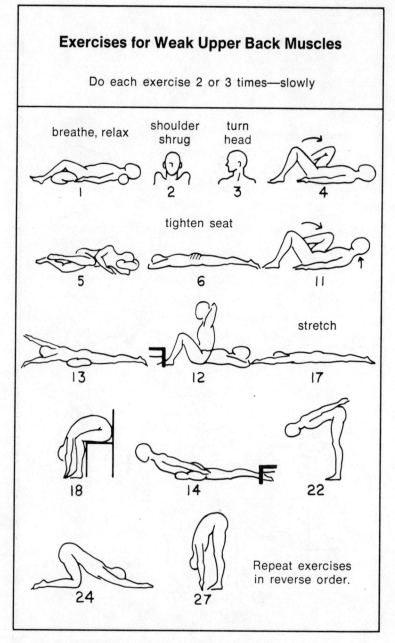

Figure 4: For Failure of Kraus-Weber Test 4

Exercises for Weak Lower Back Muscles

Do each exercise 2 or 3 times—slowly

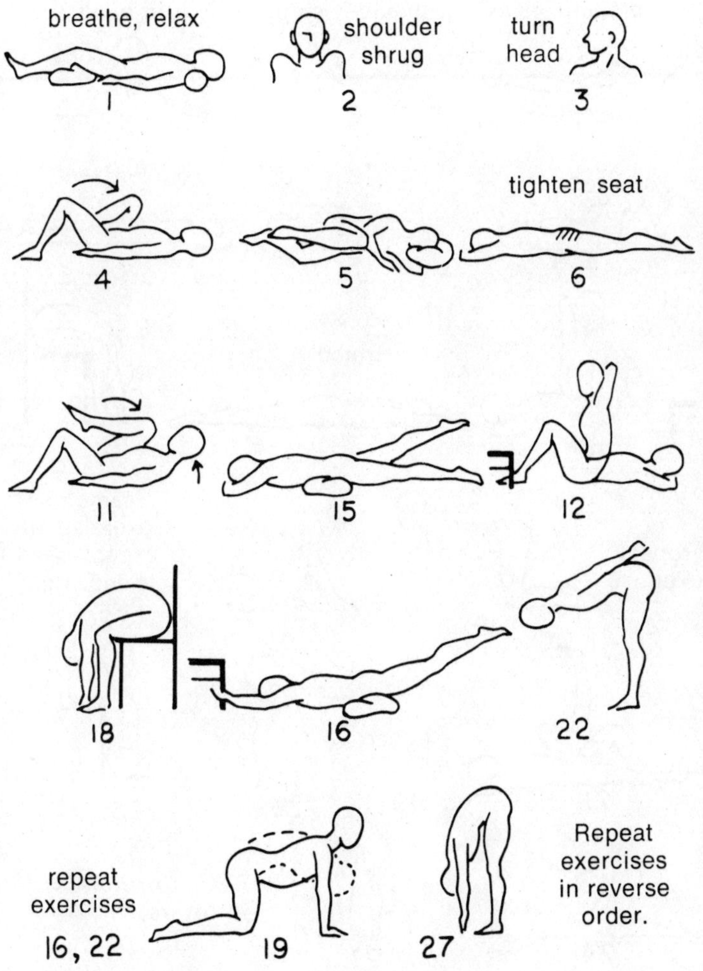

breathe, relax

shoulder shrug

2

turn head

3

1

tighten seat

4

5

6

11

15

12

18

16

22

repeat exercises

16, 22

19

27

Repeat exercises in reverse order.

Figure 5: For Failure of Kraus-Weber Test 5

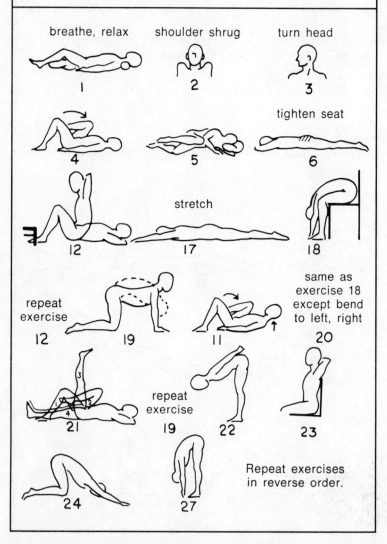

Exercises for Lack of Flexibility

Do each exercise 2 or 3 times—slowly

breathe, relax   shoulder shrug   turn head

1   2   3

tighten seat

4   5   6

stretch

12   17   18

repeat exercise

12   19   11   same as exercise 18 except bend to left, right   20

repeat exercise

21   19   22   23

Repeat exercises in reverse order.

24   27

Figure 6: For Failure of Kraus-Weber Test 6

Exercises for Weak Hip Flexing Muscles and Lack of Flexibility

Do each exercise 2 or 3 times—slowly

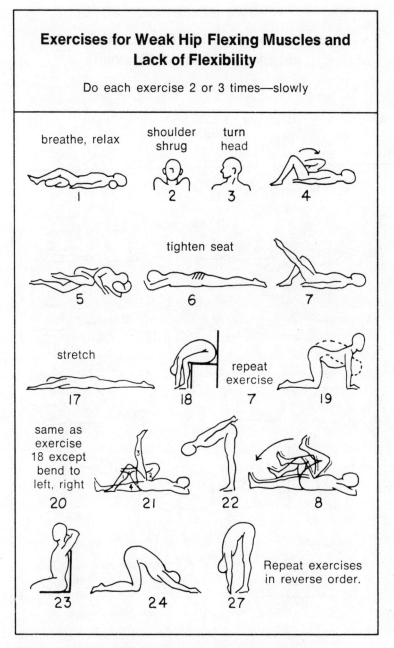

breathe, relax   shoulder shrug   turn head

1   2   3   4

tighten seat

5   6   7

stretch

17   18   repeat exercise 7   19

same as exercise 18 except bend to left, right

20   21   22   8

23   24   27   Repeat exercises in reverse order.

Figure 7: For Failure of Kraus-Weber Tests 1 and 6

Exercises for Weak Hip Flexors, Abdominal Muscles and Lack of Flexibility

Do each exercise 2 or 3 times—slowly

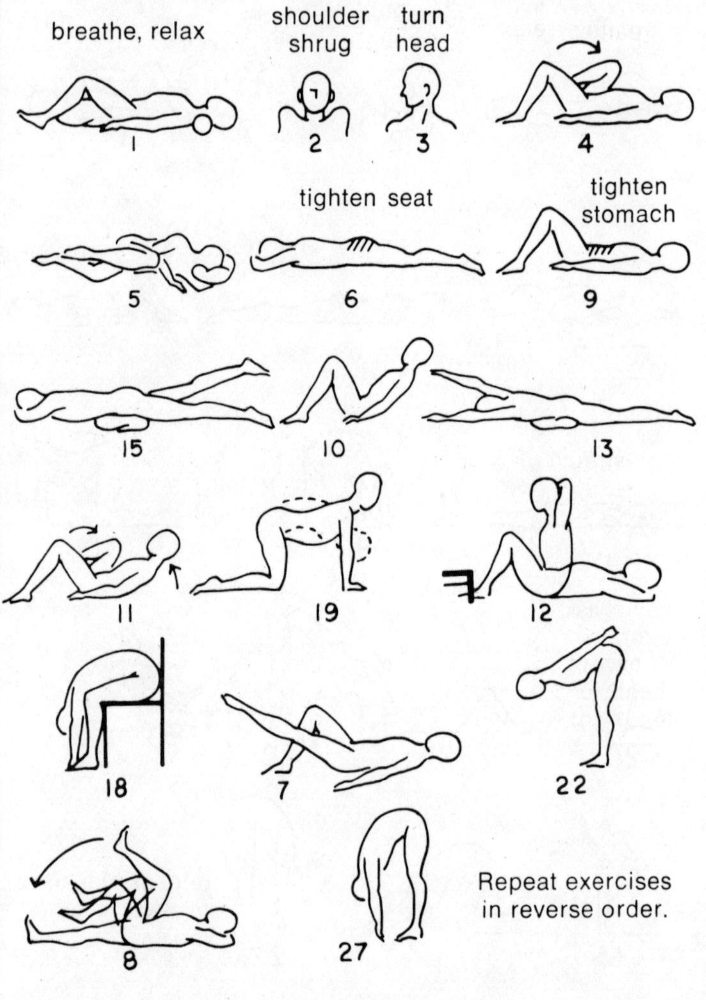

breathe, relax

shoulder shrug

turn head

1

2

3

4

tighten seat

tighten stomach

5

6

9

15

10

13

11

19

12

18

7

22

8

27

Repeat exercises in reverse order.

Figure 8: For Failure of Kraus-Weber Tests 2 and 6

Exercises for Weak Abdominal Muscles and Lack of Flexibility

Do each exercise 2 or 3 times—slowly

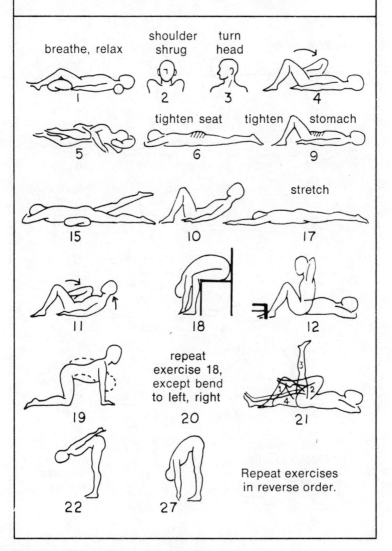

Figure 9: For Failure of Kraus-Weber Tests 3 and 6

103

Exercises for Weak Upper Back and Lack of Flexibility

Do each exercise 2 or 3 times—slowly

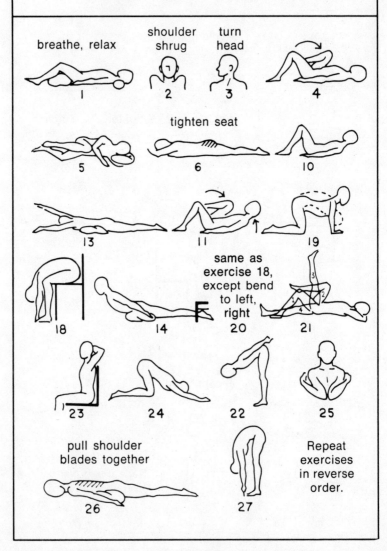

Figure 10: For Failure of Kraus Weber Tests 4 and 6

Exercises for Weak Lower Back Muscles and Lack of Flexibility

Do each exercise 2 or 3 times—slowly

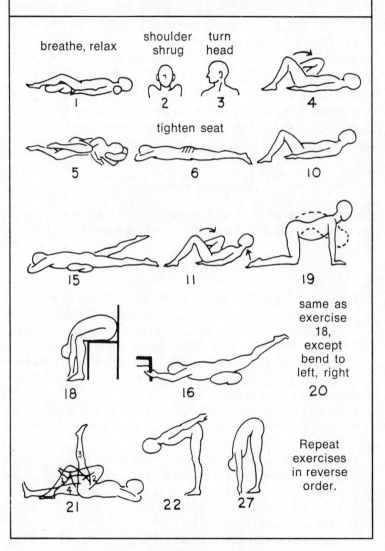

Figure 11: For Failure of Kraus-Weber Tests 5 and 6

When you feel that you are well enough to move on to some more strenuous sport, always remember to use your warming-up and cooling-down stretches before and after that activity as well. Countless joggers have injured their backs by stepping out of a hectic office and pounding the pavement without preparing the muscles. The shock can't be absorbed by tense muscles. Warm-ups stretch the tissue and make it more flexible and resilient.

If you have a back problem, be careful in choosing your sport. Obviously, tackle football is out. You might try swimming first, and then consult with your back physician about moving on to tennis or running. Whatever sport you choose, do it regularly—three or four times a week at least—to keep your muscles toned and strong.

Preventive Measures

Certain actions taken every day can put the odds in your favor against another backache. Here are some suggestions.*

Do

1. Shift your position while working in the office, at home, or driving. Standing, sitting or leaning in any position too long will make muscles tense and stiff. Try to do certain jobs in different positions every few days. Put the phone on the other side of the desk, for instance. Move around as often as you can. If you have to sit for a long time, shrug your shoulders frequently and shift in your chair every so often.
2. Sit with your feet resting on a stool to flex the knees and hips.
3. Stand with the foot on the painful side of your back resting on a stool.
4. Lie on your back with a pillow under your knees.
5. Lie on your side with a pillow between your legs.
6. Lie prone with a pillow under your hips.
7. Support your arms on a table or desk when reading.
8. Bend knees when lifting objects.
9. Sleep on a hair mattress or a latex rubber pad.

Don't

1. Crouch over a low typewriter.
2. Twist to reach the phone.
3. Cradle the phone between shoulder and ear.
4. Write under tension.
5. Read in poor light.
6. Sit in a soft chair.
7. Read in bed.
8. Stay in any frequently repeated tense, cramped position.
9. Bend from the hips.
10. Lift objects from the hips.

Restraining Treatments

We rarely advocate traction as a method of relieving back pain. Traction, or any long period of bed rest, only adds to existing muscle stiffness. In most cases, immobilization makes the backache worse than it was before the period of rest. We favor the stretching and relaxing exercises cited earlier in this chapter. In reality, these exercises are far more relaxing to the muscles than lying prone for long periods of time.

Another form of restriction is the corset that many people use after a back episode. This also prevents the muscles from getting the necessary stretch they need. We suggest the use of corsets only when a person is unable to move around without this auxiliary support. Even then, we try to treat the muscles and have such a person out of the corset at the earliest possible time.

Drugs for Back Pain

Like headaches, backaches are a leading cause of drug dependence in this country. When the pain is still intermittent, you

---

*The above lists reprinted from *Clinical Treatment of Back and Neck Pain*, 1970, with permission of Hans Kraus, M.D., and McGraw-Hill, Inc.

might take a prescribed painkiller when you have to. Then, when the pain becomes chronic, you find that you're always emptying the bottle, always tucking little foil pill packs in your pockets—panicking at the thought of being stranded somewhere with just your aching back and no capsuled comfort.

Drugs don't do a thing for your muscles. True, some relaxants can have a temporary effect on tension, but the exercise routine and trigger-point therapy are the only true methods of relieving the muscular backache.

In the treatment of backache, doctors should steer you away from drugs. They should relieve the pain by injecting or needling trigger points, by ice-massaging muscles in spasm, by regularly massaging the back and exercising it. Time and time again, this regimen is successful where all others have failed.

Surgery

As we noted throughout this chapter, 90 percent of all backaches are muscular, not caused by disk or other spinal problems. Surgery is worthless for muscular backaches. And often even disk disorders, if they're minor, will respond sufficiently to muscular therapy so that surgery can be avoided. However, some muscular conditions mimic those symptoms characteristic of a disk disorder. Because of this, many muscular back pains are diagnosed and treated as disk problems. Unless you have a severe disk disorder, recognizable by the signs given earlier in this chapter, we suggest that you seek out all forms of relaxation and muscular treatments before you go in for an operation. Remember, you have a 90 percent chance of finding relief outside the operating room.

Our research has shown us that two of the three most common chronic pains—back and head—are caused more often than not by muscle spasms, and that we can relieve the pain by treating the muscles. In the next chapter, we will discuss the third most common pain, neckache, which our research also tells us should be diagnosed and treated predominantly as a muscle-contraction disorder.

5

Your Aching Neck

Dan is dizzy all the time. When he gets up from his desk, he has to hold the back of his chair until the room stops spinning.

Fred thinks that his heart is failing. Twice this week, he's reached across his drafting board for a tool and felt a shooting pain in his chest.

Thirty-year-old Alice complains constantly about her eyes going bad at such a young age, and Sue is always leaving the office with a headache.

All these people are suffering from the same disorder: a pain in the neck. But how can a sore neck be the source of dizziness, chest pains, blurry vision and headaches? A close look at the intricate structure of the neck will give you the answer to that question.

What Causes the Pain?

Although the neck, with its forward curve and cushiony disks, was designed well to withstand shock, it is still in a vulnerable position as it balances a nine- to fourteen-pound head on its seven spindly vertebrae. Aside from this balancing act, the neck is also responsible for nodding the head, turning it from side to side, snapping it down when something flies toward the face, and all the rest of the complicated head maneuvers that allow us to seek and give information about the world surrounding us.

Almost constant head movement is made easy by the disks that lie between adjoining neck bones. These resilient pads are filled with a thick, jellylike substance. They absorb shock when we run or ride on a bumpy street as well as providing a smooth surface over which the vertebrae glide when we move our heads.

Aside from supporting the head, the neck contains many vital organs that affect the whole body. Inside the bones themselves is the spinal cord. Nerves running from the spine to the upper parts of the body, providing feeling to the arms, upper back and hands, pass through the neck bones. Each vertebra houses a nerve root which branches out to bring sensation to a specific part of the body.*

Nerve root	Skin site
C1	back of head
C2	back of head and neck
C3	upper part of neck
C4	upper shoulder and collarbone
C5	middle part of shoulder
C6	arm and hand to thumb and index finger
C7	forearm and third finger
C8	back of forearm and third and fourth fingers

Neck Nerves Which Affect Other Parts of the Body

Major blood vessels also lie in the neck, including the jugular vein and the carotid arteries, which feed the brain, face and eyes. The thyroid and other important glands are found there too, as are the throat, for food intake, and the windpipe.

Important as all these vessels, glands, nerves and passageways are to the body, they are not protected from injury by any special

*Reprinted with permission from *A Pain in the Neck,* by Ruth Winter (New York: Grosset & Dunlap, 1974).

structure such as the skull or the ribs. Sudden movements can injure the neck system. Even the stress of everyday life eventually takes its toll.

The structures in the neck that most often cause pain are the muscles. Just as in headaches and backaches, the majority of neckaches result from muscle tension. Most often, this tension is caused by one of these three factors:

Using the neck as a receptacle for stress

When a difficult situation arises, the neck muscles tighten up. If you're nodding in agreement with this statement, you can relax those muscles by consciously breaking the muscle-tension habit. When you're working at home, at school or in the office, notice your neck muscles every few hours. Do they feel tight and sore? Are your shoulders hunched up? Shrug your shoulders as high as you can and then let them go. Do a few head rolls. Sit back in your chair and take a deep breath. Exhale and let your whole body go limp. These are just a few quick exercises that will relax and loosen up tight neck muscles.

At the same time that you check your muscles for tightness, ask yourself why you are tense. Is there some irritating noise? Are you under a tough deadline? Or do you habitually tense up when you work? Keep notes on what situations cause you to tighten your neck muscles. Then, before confronting these stressful stimuli, go through a few relaxation exercises. Repeat them when the tense situation is over. (For relaxation exercises, see the following chapter.)

During a stressful period, try to break away from what you're doing and take a few deep breaths. With each one, tell yourself that you're calm. Close your eyes and relax for a moment. This break in the stress cycle takes only a few seconds, but it allows the muscles in your neck to relax and relieves some of the constant strain on them.

If you stretch the neck muscles and relax them periodically when you're under pressure, you can break the habit of tightening your neck when the heat is on.

An untreated jaw imbalance

Many neck-pain sufferers have a jaw imbalance that causes the TMJ Syndrome, described in Chapter 3. One symptom of this syndrome is neck pain caused by unusual strain on neck muscles.

When the jaw is out of balance, it alters the position of the head on the neck. The muscles supporting the head are constantly pulling and pushing the unwieldy weight to keep it balanced. Unlike emotional stress, which eases when a crisis passes, the tension caused by a jaw imbalance persists for months or years until the jaw is repositioned. Naturally, any treatment that disregarded this structural-imbalance factor would have less of a chance of success than one that addressed the widespread TMJ Syndrome.

Unfortunately, most physicians treating neck distress do not include tests for this imbalance. You can give yourself the tests described in Chapter 3 to determine the likelihood of a jaw problem. Of course, a professional diagnosis is necessary to determine the specific nature of your jaw disorder and the best way to treat it.

Poor posture habits

Tight muscles can result from poor posture as well as from emotional upset or structural imbalance. Do you sit and work with your shoulders hunched? Do you rest your head on one hand while writing? Do you prop up your head on a pillow to read or watch TV in bed? These are three of the countless familiar positions we use that are bad for the neck muscles. Some people hunch over a typewriter or ledger. Most of us crane our necks every day to shave or put on make-up. And then there's the familiar chin-shoulder sling that many of us use to keep our hands free while talking on the telephone.

Holding the neck in an awkward position once in a while won't do you any harm. But if the neck muscles are contracted in an unusual position habitually, they'll cramp up, go into spasm and cause pain. The ideal action to take is to make alterations in your environment so that you don't have to strain the muscles: Buy a shaving mirror that you can move close to your face, for instance. Unfortunately, some fixtures at home or in the office will always require neck strain. But you can be more conscious of it and keep the muscles relaxed and toned with proper exercise, as described later in this chapter.

Aside from avoiding unhealthy positions for the neck, you can also be aware of using personal effects that put stress on the neck muscles. Tight collars and thin, tight bra straps can cause problems. Foam-rubber pillows may last longer, but they don't offer the proper support provided by malleable feather stuffing. When you put your head on a foam-rubber pillow, the rubber continually bounces the head off the surface, forcing the neck muscles to work all night keeping the head down. Feathers allow the head to make an impression in the pillow at the same time that they support the nape of the neck.

Any single neck stress factor mentioned here or a combination of all three of them can start a chronic muscular disorder. At first you might not notice any discomfort. However, as the tightness persists, the muscles will be less able to stretch out to accommodate movement. One day you'll turn your head quickly to see who came in the door and the neck will go into spasm. You've doubtless seen enough comedy shows to recognize the stiff neck that results from this kind of muscle spasm. You also probably know that it's not funny when you're the person whose head is being wrenched back into position by some well-meaning, but misinformed, friend.

Pain is an obvious symptom of muscle spasm in the neck. However, many other seemingly unrelated disorders can arise from complications of the spastic muscles. The carotid arteries can be pressed, reducing the flow of blood to the brain. Faintness, vision problems, dizziness, ringing in the ears and even limb paralysis can result from the lack of blood supply. In people prone to migraine or other vascular-type headaches, this constriction of the arteries can kick off an attack.

Shooting pains into the chest and arms can occur when trigger points develop in the spastic muscles. The pains are often mistaken for heart trouble or even bursitis when the shoulder is involved.

Easing the Pain

Even when you've taken the strain off the neck muscles by correcting a jaw imbalance or altering your posture habits, your neckache may linger on until you treat the muscle spasms. After being knotted up for a long period of time, the muscles may be unable to relax naturally. And, as in any muscle-tension disorder, you'll probably have developed a few trigger points that need treatment.

The neck muscles respond to many of the treatments used for backaches. Trigger points should be injected with fluid or dry-needled to disperse them. The muscles may be sprayed with ethyl chloride or Fluorimethane, or packed in ice every few hours. Some people use moist heat rather than ice, finding that their muscles respond more to the warmth. These methods allow you to stretch and limber the muscles with the exercises given in this chapter.

Massage is also good. You must be more gentle with the neck muscles than with the back, but the same kneading, rolling motion is a good relaxer. And don't forget to massage the shoulders, upper back and arms. All the muscles in these areas will have shared the distress in the neck.

After you've lessened the pain and increased movement with the above techniques, you're ready to move on to exercise therapy, which not only relaxes and strengthens muscles, but also relieves pain and prevents future neckache episodes.

Exercises for the Neck*

Along with his exercise program for painful backs, Dr. Hans Kraus, author of *Clinical Treatment of Back and Neck Pain,* provides a daily regimen for neckache sufferers. The following routine provides you with movements to limber, relax and tone

---

*Reprinted from *Clinical Treatment of Back and Neck Pain,* 1970, with permission of Hans Kraus, M.D., and McGraw-Hill, Inc.

weak, painful neck muscles. If you work through all ten of them faithfully, the program will help you. Spotty exercising—under any circumstances—often hurts muscles more than it helps them.

The exercises should be performed in the order in which they appear. When performed from beginning to end and then in reverse, the routine provides you with warm-up movements, increasingly difficult exercises, and cool-down activities. Remember when you begin exercising that you want to stretch and tone your muscles. Rhythmic, slow movements work toward these results, while fast, jerky exertion only traumatizes the tight muscles.

To start, lie comfortably on a carpeted floor or a floor mat with a pillow under your knees, one under each of your arms, and a rolled pillow or towel under your neck. Proceed with the exercises, repeating each of them two or three times before going on to the next. Whenever you feel discomfort when you stretch, you've gone too far. Exert yourself only to the point where it starts to hurt.

1. Loosen up by wobbling your neck, shoulders, arms, thighs, legs and feet. Raise your arms slowly, then let them drop. Repeat these motions with your hands and legs and feet. Let your head drop to the left, then to the right. Take a deep breath—do not strain—exhale slowly.

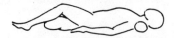

breathe, relax, turn head left, right

2. Get up, sit on a chair, shrug your shoulders.

shoulder shrug

3. Lie down. Turn your head all the way to the left, then return it to the normal front-and-center position, and relax. Turn your head all the way to the right, as far as you can, return to normal position, and relax. Also do this exercise in a sitting position.

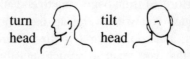

turn head   tilt head

4. Sit in a chair, place your hands behind your neck, interlace fingers. Now bring your elbows as far back as you possibly can, return to starting position, drop your arms, and relax. Repeat.

pectoral stretch, sitting

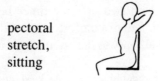

5. Sit on a chair, your hands placed on your shoulders. Try to cross your elbows by bringing your right arm as far left as possible and your left arm as far right as possible until you feel the stretch across your upper back. Return to starting position, drop your hands, and relax.

trapezius stretch

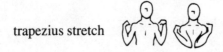

6. From a kneeling position, place your hands, then your forearms, on the floor. Gradually straighten your back, sliding forward on your arms and keeping your back and head straight. This will stretch your pectoral muscles as you move away from your knees. Return to a kneeling position, rest, and then repeat the exercise.

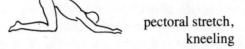

pectoral stretch,
kneeling

7. Lie on your stomach, a pillow under your hips. Pull your shoulder blades together, then relax. This exercise can be helpful in combination with the "shrugging."

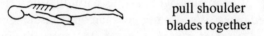

pull shoulder
blades together

8. Lie on the floor with knees flexed, hands loose by your sides. Raise your head and shoulders off the floor, bring them down slowly, and relax.

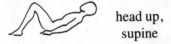

head up,
supine

9. Same as number 8, but when you raise your head and shoulders off the floor, turn your head left, then right.

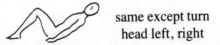

same except turn
head left, right

10. Lie on your stomach with a large pillow under your waist. Anchor your feet under a heavy piece of furniture that won't topple on you. Keeping your hands at your sides, raise your back until it is in a horizontal line—do not arch backward.

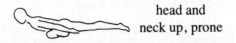

head and
neck up, prone

Drug therapy

Medicines should be used sparingly for any chronic muscular pain. You need to know how much to exercise a traumatized muscle so that you stretch it without overextending it. You need to know when the muscles begin to tense again after you've relaxed them. In the haze of narcotic painkillers, you may find it difficult to use the restorative therapies suggested in this chapter.

Non-narcotic analgesics like aspirin can be helpful in reducing pain and inflammation without the harmful side effects of more potent medicines. We also use non-narcotic muscle relaxants during the critical states of a neck disorder. However, the prescription is discontinued shortly so that the patient doesn't come to rely on a drug form of muscle relaxation. We use the medicine to help our patients advance in their exercise programs.

Recently, depression has been found to play an important role in causing chronic muscular pain. Depression and chronic headache, neckache or backache seem to go hand in hand. Unless the depression is treated, the pain often resists standard treatment methods. Our therapy often includes the use of antidepressants for a limited period of time when this disorder proves to be a component of the pain problem.

Immobilization Therapy

Cervical collars and traction can actually cause more trauma to the neck muscles rather than relieve pain. Muscular-tension disorders demand exercise to strengthen and relax tight muscle spasms. A cervical collar or a few days in traction will hold the neck rigidly in one position, causing already tense muscles to tighten up even more, thereby worsening the neck pain.

Disk Dysfunction in the Neck

Your neck is really an extension of the spine. Like the backbone, the neck consists of small triangular bones stacked on top of one another with resilient disks between them. Disk disorders are most often seen in two forms: the ruptured disk and the slipped disk.

A slipped disk occurs when a blow or sudden movement causes one or more of the pads between the vertebrae to slip out of their position, bulging between the bones and leaving too little cushioning between them.

The ruptured disk results from a blow or sudden movement also. In this disorder, the disk breaks open, allowing the thick, jellylike substance inside it to leak out into the core of the neck's vertebral column.

Muscularly, the neck stiffens to prevent further injury from movement. The slipped disk or the material that is forced out of a ruptured disk may press on the nerves in the neck, causing a numbness or tingling in the hands, arms and upper torso. The pressure on the nerves can also cause inflammation and severe pain from coughing or sudden movements. Radiating pain down the arms or into the chest is not uncommon with disk problems. We'd like to point out here that as few as one in one hundred neckaches is caused by disk damage. The rest are due to muscle spasms.

Arthritic Neckaches

Aging seems to be an easy diagnostic catchall for chronic pain problems. Unfortunately, the body doesn't retain the structural resilience that allows a child to fall down repeatedly without injury. One of the most common degenerative afflictions of the elderly is osteoarthritis: the wear-and-tear disorder. We will all suffer from it somewhere in our bodies when we grow old. As a result, the joints will become stiff and painful to move.

Whiplash

When we hear that someone is suing a driver for damages caused by whiplash, many of us will smirk and say something sarcastic about not forgetting to wear the cervical collar to court. Despite our skepticism, approximately 86 percent of car-accident victims are reported to have whiplash injuries. Usually this neck disorder will keep someone out of work for eight to ten weeks. For more severe cases, disability may last years.

Whiplash occurs most often in cars, but it can happen in any situation where the head is thrown violently forward or backward, then snaps back in the other direction. Muscles and ligaments can be torn. Disks can be forced out of position or ruptured. Even the arteries and nerves in the neck can be damaged. However, as in every other kind of neck pain, the muscles are the cause of most whiplash complaints.

The pain is almost surely muscular if the symptoms occur a few hours after the accident. The person may feel a devastating pain, usually on one side of the neck, that makes it difficult or impossible to move the head. Other common symptoms are loss of balance, headache starting at the back of the neck and radiating up the head; numbness in the extremities, usually the fingers; temporary deafness; faintness.

Since this is a muscular problem, we favor exercise as a part of the immediate treatment whenever possible. Of course, a serious injury would require a period of rest.

We have tried to show you in this chapter how exercise is a key factor in relieving chronic neck pain. This is also true in backache and headache. Exercise is good for limbering tight muscles, but new methods of relaxation make it possible to prevent muscle tightness from occurring. One of these methods is biofeedback, which we discuss in the next chapter.

6

Biofeedback: Learning to Relax

You may be familiar with the pictures of biofeedback patients laboriously wired to an alien-looking monitor, smiling beatifically with their eyes closed. Biofeedback has become synonymous with relaxation in the last decade. But in itself, it does not produce relaxation. The monitors are only an aid in learning self-induced relaxation.

Biofeedback refers to the use of muscle, temperature and brain wave monitors to quicken and deepen relaxation training. The feedback comes in the form of a needle moving back and forth, or as a sound pulse growing faster or slower. While you are monitored, the needle or sound gives you information on a moment-to-moment basis about obscure processes in the body. Using this feedback, you actually learn to control those processes that until recently were thought to be involuntary or uncontrollable. Paul Mandl, an instructor specializing in TMJ Syndrome patients, gives us his approach to biofeedback training in this discussion.

Three forms of biofeedback training are used most frequently today: muscle relaxing, blood flow control and brain wave control. The most common biofeedback programs concentrate on muscle relaxation with auxiliary blood flow control. Anyone suffering from muscle-tension pain like headaches or neckaches would most often be introduced into this program.

For migraine sufferers and victims of other disorders caused by poor circulation, temperature or blood flow control training would be indicated. If that vascular problem were mixed with muscle tension, as many neck and head aches are, you'd combine temperature and muscle-control training.

Brain wave therapy would be called for with the epileptic. Combined with muscle-relaxing biofeedback it would also be helpful for the insomniac.

No matter which biofeedback method you work with, the resultant relaxation will generalize to the rest of the body. So if you train with the muscle monitor, not only will you experience a softening of the muscle tissue, but you will also notice increasing warmth in the arms and hands, which follows temperature-control training. Your brain waves will also slow down, as they would if you were in a brain-wave-monitored biofeedback program.

These changes are all measurable and are all happening simultaneously. In biofeedback training, you emphasize one in order to gain control over all of them. We find that patients learn muscle relaxation more readily than temperature or brain wave control, so it's the method of choice. Temperature control runs a close second, however, and is often used to deepen the overall relaxation skill.

How the Monitors Work

The electromyograph (EMG) used in muscle-relaxation training is sensitive to muscle tone down to an extremely fine level. One or two muscle fibers moving would create a fraction of a microvolt. This machine is sensitive to microvolts.

An approximate guideline to monitor readings would indicate that a person in the midst of a muscle-contraction headache generally measures 20, 30, 50—even upward of 60 microvolts. A deeply relaxed person would measure about 3 or 4. And a person engaged in normal activity might measure around 15 microvolts.

These figures notwithstanding, we have had patients come in with normal activity levels of 35 to 40 who were cured of their symptoms when they dropped down to 20. Others have come in complaining of a headache at 16 microvolts and needed to relax down to 3 during sessions. Their maintenance levels were 6 or 7 microvolts.

As you can see, we're talking about a highly individual measurement. Comfort levels in the muscle are defined by many factors other than microvoltage. The biochemistry of the individual plays a part, as does his or her pain threshold. Generally, we can say that relative to each individual, you want to see the monitor indicate a proportional drop-off from the original base line to some much lower point.

Some of you may have noticed that certain biofeedback monitors are on the market for consumers. Using these monitors without the proper guidance isn't recommended by the manufacturers or by specialists in the field. You can't just hook yourself up to a monitor and make it go slower. Eventually the monitor would probably show a decrease in activity, for after thrashing around for several sessions, trying all sorts of concentration exercises or physical positions, a person would finally just give up. And when the person gives up, the monitor shows a relaxation, a lack of concentrated effort.

So you can be successful with a trial-and-error technique. But most people find it frustrating and disillusioning. The biofeedback instructor guides you quickly to your goal with specific techniques for deep relaxation. The monitor serves as an adjunct to the relaxation training. It lets you hear and see your body relaxing. You don't make the monitor slow down; you make your body loose and the monitor reflects that looseness. If the feedback shows an increase in tension, your conscious effort to bring it back down won't succeed. Nonetheless, your brain is learning what physical changes make the monitor speed up and slow down. You are involuntarily learning how to relax. But how?

In biofeedback training, we assume that initially you don't have control over physical tension. You don't know how you can create two-degree changes in your skin temperature in three minutes. Now we seat you in a comfortable chair, attach you to a monitor, and suggest that you momentarily acknowledge your desire to increase the warmth in your arms, your hands, or elsewhere in your body. You're not going to try to make them warm. You're just going to wait.

The monitor shows your temperature rising and falling off again, rising and falling. As the brain hears or sees the monitor reflecting increased warmth, it scans the whole body to see what is causing the increase. When the feedback reflects a loss of heat, the brain again scans the body to ascertain what is causing the loss. Eventually the mind will start to isolate common factors related to the needle's rise.

The practical result of this process of elimination is that while a person doesn't understand how, he or she can voluntarily warm up the hands, for instance, if the monitor is used frequently during relaxation sessions.

Put a patient on a monitor measuring fine degrees of muscle tone in the head. He or she will hear the monitor growing faster or slower, but the patient is sitting in the chair blank-faced. He or she doesn't know what is making the monitor fluctuate. The feedback reflects activity below sensation levels.

I will say to the patient, "I want the machine to read slower and more stable. Don't do anything to make it that way. Just relax and wait." After a number of sessions, the brain becomes aware of what bodily changes make the monitor speed up and slow down. The patient then will be able to walk in, sit down, and from a moderate erratic level reflected on the monitor, drop down easily to a stable and lower level.

While we have three types of biofeedback monitors—muscle, temperature and brain wave—the muscle monitor is by far the most effective for the widest range of needs. Muscle tension is fundamental to all stress problems. And when you learn to relax the muscles, the effects of that skill will generalize to all parts of the body affected by stress, like the circulatory system. You train with the muscles because they are most easily felt.

Why We Need to Relax

When we talk about muscle-tension problems, most often pain, we're talking about a habit. You learn to respond to stress with your muscles. As a child, you lived for the moment, never worrying or regretting. But as you reached age nine or ten, you became able to think backward and forward as well as about the present. You started to carry worries with you. These preoccupations—like school grades, employment, and most of all, schedules—reached down into the physical body and became tension habits.

The expression of this tension depends on the person's physical weak links. Genetically you are more prone to one kind of symptom than to another. People who have a family history of migraines are more likely to develop vascular headaches because genetically they have been dealt weak blood vessels.

A patient with a proclivity to migraines may have the same in-stream blood pressure in the brow as a non-migraineur. Yet, by genetic chance, their blood vessels are thinner-walled and more tender than those of the non-migraineur. So migraine patients will experience an attack under the same physical and psychic conditions that leave the rest of us unaffected. The migraineur is no less able to cope with a problem than we are, but physically that stress will trigger a migraine. Another person might develop an ulcer; someone else, colitis or the TMJ Syndrome.

Many times, our inappropriate tension habits develop out of a reaction to a series of real tragedies or crises. However, long after we adjust to the problems psychologically, we still use our crisis habits when relating to everyday stress.

The symptoms of our stress responses also become a way of life. We expect the symptoms to continue: "When will my next migraine come?" "I won't be able to sleep tonight." "My stomach is going to kill me after this day." In a sense, we're setting ourselves up for the pain, or the sleeplessness, or any other stress-related disorder.

In biofeedback, you learn to adjust your reaction. You learn not to become helplessly tensed up about what's happening in the world, since it's not a physical threat. You don't get a stomach ache over a deadline. You don't get a headache over the bills. The only time you become physically tense is when you're attacked by a mugger or otherwise physically threatened.

In other words, you break the cycle of tension causing pain causing more tension, etc. Once you've broken the predominant cycle, you usually won't develop another stress-related symptom.

Oh, you might have an occasional sleepless night, a stomach ache or a head pain, but you'll be able to control those isolated incidents. You'll also know that the discomfort won't be coming back again and again.

The Biofeedback Program

Before we get into the relaxation training, I'd like to mention that you don't need a biofeedback monitor to relax. You can get good results without it. However, the monitor does make your skill much more profound by extending the range of your awareness below what you can feel. And the deeper you are able to relax, the more buffered you are against symptom-level tension. The more extreme the ideal that you reach during your exercise, the better the working average is all day long.

The extra degree of refinement and sensitivity also increases your awareness when you start to tighten up. You don't go around for three hours holding yourself tense, unaware of it. Instead, you notice the tension early and let it go. You get out of trouble more quickly. Relaxation becomes much more a matter of prevention than of treatment. You don't turn off a headache; you train yourself in a habitual muscular style that precludes headaches.

The biofeedback monitor and instructor, then, will speed up the relaxation training and make it a deeply effective skill. We suggest you work with an instructor if at all possible. However, if biofeedback therapists aren't available in your area, use the guidelines that follow, the exercises at the end of this chapter, and patience and disciplined practice to create your own effective routine.

The classic program begins with a very general relaxation technique. Then, when the patient becomes skilled at this technique, we narrow in on his or her specific problem. We teach the general relaxation skill with a combination of home practice exercises and biofeedback sessions in the office. For both home routines and office visits, we use progressive relaxation. This technique requires that you mentally tune in to your body and simply become aware of how certain muscle groups feel.

Patients often notice that their muscles feel tense and then try to relax them. This is not part of the routine. Your role is purely one of passive awareness. You lie down, get comfortable, close your eyes and focus on your breathing. Again, don't try to shape your breathing pattern. Make yourself aware of its pace and depth. Observe the muscular activity when you inhale and exhale. If you try to calm your breathing, your attempts will backfire proportionately to the amount of effort you put into them. So just lie back, relax, and observe.

Following the breathing exercise, we direct the patient's attention to a series of locations in the body that are deep inside the major muscles. The patient simply notes how each location feels. He or she is not talking about it, not picturing it, not even making mental notes about each location. This is a direct sensory perception of the state of an individual muscle group. Does it feel tight? Is it relaxed? Is your impression vague? Or do you get a blank?

Whether you note tension or the lack of any sensation is unimportant. Your awareness of how the area felt, for just a moment, is the critical factor. You just catalogue the information and move on. You don't stop and say to yourself, "O.K., that's tense. Next?" Just move your attention from one location to another. Think of it as if you were asked to scan the horizon. You wouldn't stop and say to yourself, "O.K., tower, bridge, skyscraper, park." You just register the visual imagery in a clean sweep. Progressive relaxation is the sensory equivalent of a visual sweep.

We don't have to tell the body to loosen up, because the natural state of the muscles is to be soft and relaxed. Tension occurs only when you send a directive through your nervous system to brace a muscle group. You want to get away from commanding. You want to show the brain what it is like to be as relaxed as possible throughout the body. The brain already knows that you're going through these exercises to relieve tension in the body. You don't have to keep reminding yourself of that.

We have found that the deepest results come from absolutely passive awareness. That means that you're not trying to do anything—including trying to relax. Routines that require the patient to repeat, "My feet are relaxed. My legs are relaxed," and so forth are partially effective. However, they limit the depth of your training. You'll grow dependent on the inner monologue and never acquire an automatic relaxation response.

Your passive role in these exercises keeps your attention from wandering. Just as with any other skill, you'll acquire expertise if you pay attention. But with relaxation, you concentrate on doing nothing and get good results. Here's what happens: The body starts to relax. As you practice, it learns to let go. The brain is aware of some tension here and there in the overall loose body, so it has good and bad examples to follow. Naturally, the brain wants the body to be relaxed, so it will be trying to discover what makes the muscles let go.

After a number of sessions, you'll discover that without even trying to relax, you've let go after ten minutes of self-observation. The drop-off, as measured by the monitor, is often profound after just a few weeks.

The relaxation session described above usually takes eight to ten minutes. You need to practice it every day to become proficient. In our office, we devote the first four or five weeks to what we call basic training. During this time, you work with the basic relaxation technique, slightly altered from session to session, until you've cut in half the time required to run through the routine.

The first session is devoted to learning the basic technique. The second session includes working with the biofeedback monitor. Then in the next few sessions, we refine the observation skills. Instead of asking you to regard one pair of muscles, we'll ask you to be aware of two pairs. You'll become as adept at sensing four muscles as you were with two. We move from that point to awareness of six or eight muscles at a time. You'll be able to scan the entire body in one minute rather than eight. Along with the breathing exercise, your routine won't usually take more than three or four minutes.

Next, we add temperature control to the muscle sequence. Again, we ask simply that you note the changes in circulation that coincide with relaxation. You'll be aware of a decline in volume and pressure in the head at the same time that circulation increases in the arms and hands. Arms and hands will feel warm and heavy, and a sense of drainage will occur in the head.

With temperature control, autogenic phrases are quite helpful. These inner monologues use suggestion and imagery to encourage a desired effect. Autogenics make temperature control a much more friendly and cozy discipline than muscle relaxation. And that's appropriate. With muscle relaxation, your ideal is to feel nothing when you do the observation exercises. You want to feel a lack of tension or sensation. With circulation awareness, you're looking for certain additive sensations—warmth in the arms, a tingling in the neck or face as circulation declines there, and heaviness in the arms and hands. So you can use positive, suggestive imagery and it will be productive.

For instance, you might want to use phrases like: "I feel my arms and hands becoming warmer." Or you might choose a situational suggestion like the following one: You're on a terrace at the beach. A gentle sea breeze is blowing in and it's about 89 degrees and sunny. You're seated at a white enamel table shaded by an umbrella. While your hands are resting on the edge of the table, baking hot, your head is shaded by the umbrella.

Absolutely every sensation in that image is applicable to your sensations during the temperature-control exercise. Of course, this imagery is just an aid. You can use it to help you start feeling the circulation changes inherent in relaxation, but it's better to forgo the visualization once you've become proficient at altering the blood flow. The reason, again, is to avoid becoming dependent on the suggestion. If you need the serenity of a beach scene to relax, you'll find it tough to do so in a traffic jam or on the subway—when you need to most.

If you work through your routine once a day, you'll become a talented relaxer after four or five weeks. When you take the time to lie down or sit back comfortably at your desk, you can let go completely. Unfortunately, when you get back into daily activity, you'll be as tense in five minutes as you were before the session. So our next step in training is to make your relaxation skill an all-day habit. That's the second half of the program, and it takes several weeks.

How do you become habitually relaxed? More specifically, how can you use your relaxation skill to rid yourself of symptoms? These talents go hand in hand. In other words, if you're not continually tensing your muscles, you won't suffer the chronic ailments of strained muscles.

The first step toward generalizing your skill is to take your ability to relax deeply at will and spread its effects over the entire day. We use a brief, simple technique of releasing to achieve this. In ten to twenty seconds, you take three breaths, each one becoming gently deeper than the previous one. On each breath, you tune into a different part of your relaxation program. During the first breath, you recall the overall effect of the routine on your body—the profoundly limp, slack, loose level you can attain. And in one breath, you have let go toward that ideal state. Of course, you can't relax that deeply in a moment, but that's what you aim for.

In the second breath, you select a tense muscle to work on. Maybe it's in your neck, or your jaw, or the shoulder area. Whatever the muscle, you imagine it draining and becoming softer during the second breath.

Finally, on your third breath, you imagine that your hands have already become warm and heavy.

This exercise extracts the three principal properties of your long routine: the muscle looseness, the overall slackness, and temperature control. The key to this release break is the first breath; you're remembering to let go. You can change any habit, like a stress response, by frequent repetition of a new correct behavior. It's not very interesting or intellectually stimulating, but plugging away at the same practice routines, day after day, is the only way to alter behavior. There are no shortcuts.

Because this exercise is boring, easy to forget, we usually pick a cue or trigger peculiar to your milieu that will remind you to release. A man who runs a retail store will release to the register bell. A secretary who types letters all day will let go with every "Yours truly." If you have to wait for an elevator every day, pause and relax. When you dial someone on the phone, release while you wait for them to answer. At a red light, let go. We have tons of empty moments in our days during which we could do this release exercise without interrupting a schedule.

You do the release exercise independently of whether you need to or not. The release trigger might go off when you notice that you're already loose and relaxed. But let go anyway, so that relaxing becomes reflexive. You actually undermine the existent tension habit by letting go again and again and again. You're physically memorizing the release skill.

The second step in generalizing your relaxation focuses your skills on minor, but specific, problems. You might use the release exercise before seeing someone who gets on your nerves. Maybe you can use it for activities to which you have an aversion—say, giving speeches at a club of which you've been inadvertently elected treasurer. Driving through the city might bother you. You don't want to pick some monumental crisis or your original symptom for this stage of the training. You want an event that is recurrent, obnoxious and predictable, so that you can practice against it.

Our aim in step two is to start you using your skill specifically to relax into a problem. Tension is highest during the anticipation of some difficult circumstance. Rather than going in fighting, we want you to "release" into these minor traumas.

Usually our patients make a catalogue of situations that annoy them. Then they choose one or two of these situations and become desensitized to them. After a while, the relaxation skill becomes an automatic circuit breaker. By the time you sit down to relax, you're already calm. You might think: Why did I ever bother to get upset about this anyway? It's not worth it. So the training process becomes more of an insight than an exercise.

In the final stages of application, we zero in on whatever physical symptoms remain. Usually the patient reports few if any episodes of his or her original complaint. And when a symptom does appear, it's usually mild and manageable. All the previous training has started to change the underlying stress habits that culminated in a headache, a neckache or another disorder.

When the symptom does occur, we encourage the patient to hesitate before popping a painkiller or tranquilizer. He or she should stop the immediate activity, lean back, and relax. Remember, tension over discomfort only compounds the pain. If you can break the cycle, you stand a chance of relieving the symptom. So use the relaxation techniques; go through your routine right there in the office or at home. You may find that the pain dissipates to the point where you won't need any medication. Perhaps the first few times you try using relaxation to rid yourself of some tension complaint, you'll need the added benefit of a drug. But if you routinely approach the pain with your exercises, you'll increase their effectiveness in turning off the discomfort.

Do I Have to Do This Forever?

No. Most of our patients finish this three-part course in three or four months. At that point you don't have your original symptom; you don't carry tension around with you any longer. You'll also find that sleeping is easier and better, fatigue is no longer a problem, and you have more patience—a better perspective on your life. Of course, if you start to feel some of those old physical stress-related habits returning, you can take a short refresher course to reestablish the skill.

Does Biofeedback Work for Everyone?

Just about every human being has the potential to train in biofeedback—that is, physically. We find that the obstacles to overcome are psychological. In fact, you can break the patient population into two groups: one that will most often be successful in relaxation training, and one that will predictably resist it.

The successful group we call internalizers. These people believe that they have the last word in what happens to them. They are self-reliant and self-motivated, which is important in biofeedback training. We don't do anything to you. In the discussion of the program, you didn't see any section where the instructor talked you into relaxing. The patient is doing all the work. Unless he or she has the desire and the discipline to take the necessary time and plug away at the exercises, a patient will never become adept at this skill. So the patient who wants to change and believes that he or she can alter stress behavior will become a talented relaxer.

The unsuccessful group is the externalizers. They feel that the world happens to them. Tragedies befall them, headaches, neck-aches and fatigue plague them, and doctors cure them. These patients come into the biofeedback course much as they would go in for surgery or to a chiropractor. They want it done to them. They want to be made relaxed. For those patients, the power of muscular release lies in the monitor or in the instructor. And as you can see from our discussion here, that's simply untrue.

The externalizer will come in for session after session and complain that nothing is happening. He or she becomes frustrated and resentful, believing that the instructor is holding out on the promised cure. Unfortunately, until this person makes the psycho-logical step over to self-control, this skill will never be mastered.

Next we have the neurotic patient who doesn't really want to be healthy. He or she revels in some secondary gain of the chronic disorder. Perhaps social pressures have been lifted. Maybe financial responsibilities have been assumed by another member of the family. Or maybe the attention paid to this patient by the family on account of his or her illness is hard to let go of. Obviously, if a person doesn't want to learn the relaxation talent, for whatever reason, you can't force the issue. So the patient who wants to stay sick rarely succeeds in this training.

Finally, we come to age. It's the unfortunate truth that the older you are, the less susceptible you are to biofeedback training. Your habits are more firmly ingrained as each year passes. It's far easier to tell a sixteen-year-old adolescent to concentrate on doing nothing than it is to tell a fortyfive-year-old executive.

We might ask that executive, for instance, to increase his or her awareness from a pair of muscles to two pairs. At the next session, the patient most likely will say, "Wow, this was a tough week. You know, it's hard enough trying to relax two muscles at a time, but when you try to relax four . . ." It's as if we never said, "Don't try anything; just catalogue impressions." For these people, the training can be frustrating, actually doing more harm than good if the patient gets wound up about not being able to relax.

Exercises to Do at Home

These techniques, designed by biofeedback instructor Paul Mandl, can help you learn physical relaxation—first as a conscious skill, and finally as an automatic habit. Actually, your current stress responses and stress-related symptoms are, themselves, *learned bad habits*. The following techniques can help you learn to unlearn those stress-response habits and acquire a *naturally relaxed physical style*.

Learning physical relaxation is just like learning to drive a car or serve a tennis ball: it is a matter of following some appropriate techniques, repeating them frequently, and letting your body gradually adopt these techniques as built in. Notice that in learning a physical skill, you don't have to understand exactly *how* your nerves and muscles learn. All you have to do consciously is keep practicing the correct techniques and be aware of the results of each effort. The appropriate trend will automatically follow—that is, your skill will gradually improve.

Since the process of learning relaxation as a physical style is really the process of unlearning your stress habits, the most important ingredient in this process is *becoming aware of your stress habits* (for example, chronic scalp muscle tension leading to headaches). This awareness is the *main objective* to the following routines. As you increase your conscious awareness of even your most subtle stressful behaviors, *your mind and body will automatically begin to change their behavior in order to feel better*. Your nerves and muscles will gradually reduce their stress-response habits. You will actually be learning to adjust your own physiology to a healthier style.

So your principal role in these techniques is to learn physical self-awareness, to become more and more attuned to the obvious *and* subtle states of your body. As a result, these techniques do not include a lot of the suggestive and hypnotic language you will find in many published relaxation procedures. Such procedures *can* help you relax, but only if you have the time and place to go and perform them, quietly and alone. Unfortunately, you probably find yourself tense, and wishing you could relax, in just those situations that don't permit you to go off and be alone with your relaxation technique.

In contrast, the skills described below are designed to teach you how to be naturally relaxed by habit, instead of how to get relaxed only after you're already tense. Eventually it becomes no longer necessary to practice these techniques at all.

Finally, these techniques are based on the successful stress-relief training of thousands of medical and dental patients. The general principles behind the routines are true for all people. But you as an individual will have your own specific reactions while learning them. If you find certain variations from the exact patterns described below appear to work better for you—that is, seem more effective—then feel free to follow your body's inclinations. Basically, follow the prescribed routines as closely as possible, but when it comes down to small details, do what you discover seems to work best for you.

Planning Your Self-Awareness Training

The techniques below are labeled as follows:

> PHAT—Physical Habit Awareness Techniques
> MAP—Muscle Awareness Pattern
> CAP—Condensed Awareness Pattern
> CAT—Circulation Awareness Technique
> EAR—Exhale-Aided Releases
> SHOP—Sleep Habit Optimization Process
> POD—Process of Desensitization

Of course, these labels are for convenient reference, but in reality your learning experience will not occur in clear separate steps. Instead, one level of learning will blend into the next; your skill in one technique will continue to improve while you begin to practice the next.

The following schedule is suggested for acquiring the fullest benefits of each stage of training. *Do not* be in a hurry to "achieve." You cannot make the mind/body change its style in a day or a week; you cannot force this learning to happen faster by "trying harder." *Repetition* and *time* are the ingredients for effective and durable changes in physical habits. So *focus* on the following techniques *correctly*, do them *consistently, be patient,* and let the *powers of time and repetition* bring about the inevitable results for you.

Try to keep to the following schedule as closely as possible. On the other hand, you should feel completely familiar with each level of technique before proceeding to the next. So if necessary, continue for a few extra days or a week with any given level, until you feel "at home" with it. Then begin the next stage of the program:

Starting today, and throughout training	Practice all PHAT, incl. "Posture" and "Movement"
Week 1	Practice MAP, 1–2 times a day
Week 2	Practice CAP, 1–2/day
Week 3	Practice CAP + CAT, 1–2/day
Weeks 4–5	Practice CAP + CAT, 1/day
	Use EAR, 10–20/day
Weeks 6–7	Practice CAP + CAT, 3–4/week
	Use EAR, 10–20/day
	Begin SHOP, at each sleep
Weeks 8 and thereafter, as necessary	Practice CAP + CAT, 1–2/week
	Use EAR, at your discretion
	Continue SHOP, at each sleep
	Begin POD, as needed

All practice and application techniques are to continue until no longer needed. You'll know when this is, because your stress symptoms will be eliminated, or at least minimized, and you'll find you have a generally increased feeling of internal calm and well-being.

PHAT
(PHYSICAL HABIT AWARENESS TECHNIQUES)

Common bad habits

Starting right away, try to become conscious of *any* of your physical habits (postures or movements)—especially in the head, neck or shoulder areas. Make a written list of those you already know of, and add to that list each habit you discover from now on. Ask family members and friends to help you compile the list.

Then begin to eliminate these habits one by one. If necessary, use notes and signs to yourself. Ask others to remind you, matter-of-factly, without opinion, each and every time they see you repeating your habit(s). By these methods, you should gradually be able to let go of all those common muscular behaviors that have no positive value anyway, and are definitely harmful to your situation, such as:

Very damaging habits

- frowning steadily (aside from expressing yourself in conversation)
- clenching your teeth when angry or anxious
- working at a surface that's too high for you
- slouching into an armchair, or placing your elbows so that your shoulders are elevated above their natural hanging position
- watching TV (or anything else) with your head at a sharp angle—for example, lying in bed with your chin on your breastbone
- hunching your shoulders against cold weather or chilly rooms (use warm neckwear, and let your shoulders hang loosely)

Moderately bad habits

- biting your fingernails or lips
- chewing on pens, pencils, etc.

- supporting a pipe with teeth instead of hand
- resting your chin on your hand(s)
- tilting your head and twisting your hair with your fingers
- driving with your shoulders held up, even slightly
- standing with all your weight on one leg
  . . . and many others.

Probably the most common and injurious muscular habits are *facial tensions* and *shoulder hunching*. Like all tension habits, they usually go on unconsciously for many years, so they are not easy to get rid of quickly. But you can *gradually learn* to stop doing them, by repeatedly noticing them and letting them go.

So every time you pass a mirror, and have even a few seconds to spend, stop, look yourself full in the face, and let all your facial muscles fall slack—jaw, brow, etc.

Make sure, no matter what you're doing, that your shoulders are hanging in place. This means, when you're sitting in an armchair, place your elbows so that your shoulders are hanging limp, not propped up. And—very important!—check the height of all desks, tables, countertops and other working surfaces where you spend time: they should be low enough in front of you so that—as you work at them with your hands—your albows are at no less than a right angle, 90 degrees. If you have to raise your forearms higher than that in order to work at that surface, then your hands will be awkwardly positioned and your shoulders will unconsciously rise to compensate. So if necessary, raise the chair or lower the work surface.

Also, watch yourself while driving. You'll find you *can* drive with your shoulders hanging relaxed, and still have a safe, firm grip on the steering wheel.

Breathing style

Nothing is more important for relaxing your physical style—and generally improving your well-being—than the way you breathe.

Therefore, as often as you can remember to, *take notice of how your breathing feels*. Take a couple of fuller breaths if you like, but then let your breathing settle into its own natural shape and speed. The *size* of each breath is not as important as its *shape*. Your stomach should swell at the beginning of each inhale—this means your *diaphragm* is pulling the air deep down into the lungs, as it is supposed to do. Don't expand your chest or lift your shoulders. When exhaling, don't push the air out; just let the weight of your chest fall by itself, and notice there is a natural pause between the end of each exhale and the beginning of the next inhale.

Of course, you can *experiment* with all kinds of breathing patterns:

- holding inhales a moment before exhaling
- breathing in through the nose, out through the mouth
- counting systems (e.g.—silently counting up to 5 while inhaling, back down to zero while exhaling, etc.)
- closing your eyes, imagining you are breathing the air *into yourself through certain points,* such as the stomach surface, the middle of your chest, the nose, the center of your brow, the top of your head
- shaping each breath into a wave, filling the lungs from the bottom upward, like a sack filling with liquid, so the inhale feels as if it grows from the diaphragm upward through the lungs to the throat in an expanding wave

Try anything you like; *use anything that feels good.*

But basically, for a good general breathing style, let your diaphragm/stomach start each inhale, pulling the air into the lower end of your lungs.

Posture

In order to discover, and gradually acquire, the *optimum posture for your body* (the posture that will allow you to feel better and look your best), simply pause occasionally each day and do the following:

Stand comfortably erect. Gently but firmly roll your shoulders upward and backward, until they feel stretched to a comfortable limit. Pause. Then simply let them fall (completely unaided) down into a passively hanging position. If this doesn't feel entirely natural to you, that's only because you are not used to this posture—your nerves and muscles just aren't familiar with the feel of it. But it *is* a healthy posture for you, and by practicing it repeatedly, you *will* eventually become familiar with it—it *will* feel natural.

Now, with your shoulders dropped correctly into place, adjust your head's position as follows: keeping your eyes straight ahead and your head level, slide your head gently backward on your neck as far as possible without squeezing your throat uncomfortably. Next, tip your head back a little, and *very gently* let it rock slightly in all directions (side to side, front to back, very small circular rotations). Carefully sense the feeling of the weight of your head resting evenly on your neck, like a bowling ball balanced delicately on a small cushion. Now let your head tilt forward again to a level position.

Finally, imagine a string extending from the ceiling (or sky) down just exactly to the middle of the top of your head. The purpose of this string is to remind you not to droop or slouch down out of this optimum posture that you're learning.

Movement

When you've adjusted your head and shoulders as described above, take a full breath (expanding your stomach and chest, *not* raising your shoulders). Now, as you release the breath, imagine your "center of gravity" (a feeling like the middle of all your weight) sinking slowly down through your stomach and gently settling in the pit of your abdomen. Repeat this once or twice, and you will discover a sense of standing stable and relaxed, with your weight holding you close to the floor or ground, your shoulders and head tall and graceful like a dancer's.

Now, when you move, concentrate on the motion of that center of gravity in the pit of your abdomen. Imagine that your legs, arms and head are merely extensions of your trunk, and that basically it's your trunk (especially that center of gravity) that's moving from one place to another. This way, you can feel yourself move with a graceful, almost effortless style. Don't worry about this style of movement feeling "put on" and self-concious—after all, it does look better and feel better, and it will come to feel natural with practice.

Finally, when using your arms and hands for anything, make a habit of using the *smallest necessary muscles* for the task you're performing. For example, dial a telephone by loosely swiveling your hand only up to the wrist; you shouldn't need to move your arm or shoulder at all.

Start noticing how you carry out all arm and hand activity: If the fingers will do it, leave the arm still; if the arm can handle it, let the shoulder hang loose and still; and so forth. Don't use more muscles than are truly necessary for the comfortable, accurate performance of whatever you are doing.

Together with the released breath, lowered center of gravity, comfortably hanging shoulders and balanced head, this practice of using the *least necessary muscle power* and *fewest necessary muscles* will lead to several valuable changes in your physical experience. You will be moving less of your weight, using less muscle overall, and therefore *expending less energy* than before for the same activities. Also, when you move a smaller part of your body, you can move it *more accurately* than a larger part of you. The gradual but inevitable results will be reduced tension and fatigue, increasing energy, grace of movement and sense of well-being.

MAP
(MUSCLE AWARENESS PATTERN)

This technique will develop your *awareness of your larger muscles*. This is a physical *skill-learning* procedure—not self-hypnosis, and not fantasizing. So let yourself be physically passive, but mentally aware and alert.

At first, you will practice this awareness self-consciously at certain times; then gradually it will become automatic, unconscious and continuous—in other words, *habitual*. Furthermore, this *mus-*

cle awareness is really all that's necessary in order for your brain's muscle-control centers to learn deep relaxation! Also, since muscles comprise a large portion of your body weight, learning to let *them* relax will lead to relaxation of your entire system.

For the first couple of practice sessions, you may have someone read the techinque aloud to you, slowly, one sentence at a time, followed by ten- to fifteen-second pauses. The reader should omit the sentences indented below—as long as *you* have already read them, completely understand them, and follow their principles in your own mind.

Beginning with the third or fourth practice, you should experience the technique on your own—as best you can remember it in your own mind. Don't be too concerned about precision, or remembering exactly every sequence of details. Instead, focus on adopting the correct general style of the technique.

In the earlier weeks of practicing relaxation techniques, use common sense to avoid unnecessary distractions. For example, (1) practice in a room alone, without any background radio or music; (2) arrange to have someone else answer the phone, if convenient, or take it off the hook during your practice; (3) don't practice when you're in a hurry, or due to leave for an appointment soon; (4) to avoid drowsiness, do not practice in the late evening or right after meals.

If you do find yourself getting sleepy while practicing a routine, then try one or more of the following:

1. Temporarily open your eyes, stretch your arms and take a couple of full breaths; then resume the routine.
2. Practice during daylight, if possible.
3. Keep lights on bright instead of dim.
4. Practice in a sitting or semi-reclined position.
5. Vary the sequence of the muscle locations you focus on; for example, proceed from head to toe.
6. Shift your focus from one location to another more quickly than usual, and repeat the entire sequence a second time through.

Technique

Lie down on your back on a carpet or rug, your heels several inches apart and your feet falling naturally to the sides. Let your arms lie out from your body at a comfortable angle—palms up or down, whatever's natural for you. Make any small adjustments in your hips, shoulders, neck and head until you feel as completely as possible "sunk into the floor."

> With a few days' practice, you'll find this position more naturally and automatically comfortable. Use small pillows under your neck and lower back only if absolutely necessary.

Now close your eyes and slowly take a couple of deeper breaths. Begin to focus all your attention on *how your breathing feels*. *Do not try to control the breathing pattern,* but *simply become aware* of any or all of the following:

- the rise and fall of the chest and stomach
- the slight stretching and loosening of some chest and rib-cage muscles with inhale and exhale
- the small pause between each exhale and inhale
- the flow of air into the nose and throat (cool) and back out again (warm)
- how far down into the lungs the air is flowing
- whether the depth of breathing seems full or shallow
- whether the rhythm of the breathing seems uneven or regular
- any other physical sensations of the breathing process that you become sensitive to

After a short time, your breathing will settle into a comfortable, steady, relaxed rhythm, and will no longer feel self-conscious, even though you are observing how it feels. It will seem to be a physical process that is happening naturally—that you're conscious of, but not interfering with. Continue this focus for another moment or so.

Now begin to focus in each of the muscle locations listed below, beginning with the centers of your left and right arches.

Do not move or contract the muscles in order to feel them better. *Don't* try to picture them in your mind. *Don't* recite this routine in your mind. *Do not try to relax* the muscles you're focusing in.

Do not even "try to feel" the muscles themselves. *Simply direct your attention*—focus all your awareness—into each location for a long, quiet moment. If there is any sensation to feel, you'll feel it without trying to.

For example, you may be aware of stiffness or tightness in the muscle location in which you're focusing. This feeling can be quite subtle. Or perhaps the location feels clearly relaxed, warm, comfortable, even slightly tingling. Or maybe you have a vague sense that the flesh actually *exists* at that location, but nothing clearer than that. Or you could sense *nothing at all*—literally as if there's thin air where that part of your body should be. In any case . . .

It does not matter what impression you get of each location as you come to focus in it (tense or relaxed, clear or vague or blank). *It only matters that you quietly, effortlessly focus in each place long enough* (several breaths will usually do it) *to become aware of it as a location,* to become conscious of any slight or subtle feeling, if there's any at all.

Don't be concerned if the left and right locations of a pair of muscles feel different in any way. One may be clearer to you than the other, or more tense, for example. Left-right differences are quite common.

And *very important,* do not be concerned about mental distractions—for example, finding that your mind has wandered off to other thoughts. Distractions will happen anyway, *so no matter how often* it happens, each time you become aware that you're distracted from the routine, *simply return your attention* to the point in the routine where you were last focusing.

Also, don't bother trying *not* to think of other things, or trying *not* to visualize the muscles, or trying *not* to hear outside sounds, or trying *not* to be sleepy, or trying *not* to feel pain that you may have. You can't block things out of your mind. You can't cancel these distractions anyway, so just keep returning your attention to the muscle-location awareness pattern.

Now shift your attention from the arches to your right and left calves. Imagine a point deep inside the center of each calf muscle and become conscious of those two locations. Be aware of the pressure of their contact with the floor. The muscles may feel soft and sunk into the floor, or stiff and pressing against it. This will probably become as clear as it can ever be, within the space of several breaths.

Now continue this style of awareness in the following locations—one pair of points, or one area, at a time—focusing deep inside the centers of each muscle:

- arches
- calves
- middle of thighs
- hips or buttocks
- palms, or balls of thumbs
- thick upper portion of the forearms
- middle of each upper arm
- outside corner of each shoulder
- stomach surface, or front abdominal muscles
- chest surfaces and rib-cage (slightly stretching and loosening with the breathing)
- lower back muscles (arched stiffly off the floor, or sunk down into it?)
- upper back muscles (feel the pressure of contact with the floor)

- base, back and sides of the neck
- jaw hinges
- cheeks
- eyes, especially deep inside them
- brow
- temples
- scalp

Awareness of some muscles can sometimes be very subtle, but be patient. Direct your attention to *each* of these locations in this outline *every* time you experience the routine. Remember, it is not necessary to feel anything clearly in any given location, on any given day. It's only important to direct your attention to each location in its turn. It is the *method* that matters, not the "results." The value of orienting yourself to the *technique of awareness* (rather than the results of each separate observation) will become clearer to you after you've been experiencing this routine for a couple of weeks. Meanwhile you may be surprised at how relaxed you become by the end of a practice session—*even though you were not consciously trying to relax.*

Now return your attention to your breathing. Become as fully aware of its sensations as you were at the beginning of the routine.

In addition, become generally aware of the condition of your four limbs—whether they feel heavy, limp, sinking into the floor; or light, floating, even missing completely; warm or cool, at the skin surface or deep inside; tight or loose; etc.

Become conscious of the entire length of your back, from the lower spine through the mid and upper back to the base of the neck. Be aware of whether the length of your back feels generally stiff and pressing against the floor; or soft and sunk into the floor, as if melted into it.

Become conscious of the surfaces of your head and your facial features—the degree to which they feel blank, slack, drained, empty, expressionless, like a lifeless mask.

Now for the next few moments, plan on changing nothing at all—no stretching, no deeper breathing, no shifting or fidgeting or any other voluntary movement. *Leave everything exactly as it is.* But simply let your eyelids flip open so you can see the room above and around you.

At this moment you may feel a little disoriented. The room may seem "dreamlike," or your body may feel "unreal." This is a typical (and harmless) reaction in the first week or two, especially when the practice has been a good one (clearly felt and deeply relaxing).

> This physical state, this moment of total physical passiveness but with the eyes open, sets a very important example for the brain. It demonstrates that you can think, hear, and even *see*, without the use of any muscles. It shows that you can be completely relaxed physically while mentally aware and attentive. After a week or so of practice, it will no longer feel strange to you.

Finally, when you wish, take a couple of deeper breaths, slowly get up, and go about your next activity. As you do this, keep remembering how you felt just before, and just after, opening your eyes at the end of the routine. Especially keep in mind that feeling of looseness in your muscles and slackness in your face. Try to leave your body in that condition as continuously as possible.

CAP
(CONDENSED AWARENESS PATTERN)

In practicing the first week's routine (MAP), you've found that—at least in privacy—a simple, effortless pattern of muscular self-awareness can lead to a deeply relaxed state. But the ultimate purpose of this training program is to become able to release tension, to calm the body at will, even in difficult, real-life circumstances. So the next step in your training is to learn how to tune in to your muscles more and more quickly.

You will find that as you learn to sense all your muscles more swiftly—but still very clearly—then that familiar relaxed state comes more and more quickly too. Eventually you will be able to call upon this ability in just a moment's time, wherever you are, whenever you need it. As in the case of any physical skill, it's only a matter of practicing the right techniques often enough.

For example, a tennis player may spend hundreds of hours practicing how to serve—studying the details of racket grip, stance, balance, motion, timing, ball toss, and so forth. But after months of practice, when this player competes in a match, *he just serves*. He doesn't think of details; he can't, because of time and pressure; he justs lets his body automatically carry out the complex serving motion as one smooth, integrated, quick action. Of course, it's not perfect every time, but it's pretty reliable, and it continues to improve with practice.

Now, the same principles apply to learning how to relax, even in busy, demanding situations. In fact, being relaxed is a much simpler skill than serving a tennis ball. It only *seems* difficult because you've never really spent time *practicing* relaxation, and you've never had the appropriate instruction before. So follow these routines, and your detailed practice techniques will gradually integrate into a quick, effective skill.

Here, then, is how to begin condensing the MAP into the CAP:

Begin your practice routine as usual. Settle into position on the floor, close your eyes, focus on your breathing a minute or two, and then direct your attention to the centers of your arches. After a moment, when you are as aware of those spots as possible, shift your attention to the centers of your calves, as usual.

Now return your attention to your arches, and regain your awareness of them for a moment. They should come clear for you almost immediately, since you were just focusing in them a few moments ago, before the calves. Now return your attention to the centers of your calves, until they're clear again. And then the arches once more, until they're clearly felt. Then the calves again. And so forth, alternating your focus of awareness several times from one pair of muscle locations to the other.

Now repeat this pattern of focusing with each of the following combinations. Become clearly aware of one pair of locations (or area), then the next pair (or area), then alternate several times between being clearly aware of one and then the other.

arches . . . . calves
backs of thighs . . . . fronts of thighs
palms . . . . forearms
upper arms . . . . surfaces of the shoulders
stomach surface . . . . chest and rib cage
lower back . . . . upper back
back of the neck . . . . sides of the neck
jaw hinges . . . . cheeks
eyes
brow . . . . temples . . . . scalp

Then complete the routine as always, with whole-body awareness and eye opening without movement.

This alternating-focus technique will gradually lead to changes in how you feel your muscle locations. As you practice each day, you'll begin to find that you feel groups of four muscle spots (for example, both arches and both calves) simultaneously, but separately and clearly. Of course, the different locations within a group may not all feel the same; but you will begin to find yourself conscious of four places at once, without even trying to be.

Similarly, muscular areas (such as the stomach and chest) will seem to merge into larger areas (for example, the entire front surface of your trunk, from pelvis to collarbones).

Some of these combinations or blends will develop clearly sooner, some in later practices. As each group or larger area begins to come clearly and effortlessly for you, during several successive practice sessions, then you can stop using the alternating approach for that group or area. Simply focus into the whole combined group or larger area when you come to it in each practice from then on.

Within a week or two, most or all of these combinations or blends should have merged pretty clearly for you. At that point, you see, you will be focusing in half as many sets of muscles as before, but twice as many muscles at a time. Yet the clarity of details of your awareness, your quality of focus in each muscle of each group, should be equal to the clarity you experienced in the initial, uncondensed MAP pattern.

As it is with practicing anything consistently, your mind will get quicker and clearer and more consistent in its ability to focus through the sequence of muscle groups. And of course, now you'll be focusing into more muscles at a time. As a result, you'll find this routine beginning to take less and less time than it used to.

On the other hand, remember, don't hurry it, and don't drag it out. Always let the routine take *just the time it needs* to be effortless, clear and methodical. Continue to enjoy the routine as a sensory experience, rather than treating it as a precision drill to be performed correctly. Let yourself be absorbed in the process, the style of the routine, rather than being concerned about "results." If you simply pay attention to following these techniques in the manner described for you, you will find that "results" follow gradually and surely. You never have to try for them.

CAT
(CIRCULATION AWARENESS TECHNIQUE)

The Circulation Awareness Technique is designed to help you feel changes that occur in your blood vessels as you become more relaxed. These sensations are completely natural ones, so though they may seem strange to you at first, don't be concerned if it takes a few times for you to get used to them.

This sequence is to be followed directly *after* you reach the end of your Muscle Awareness Pattern (MAP), and *before* you open your eyes to end the practice routine.

While the MAP is strictly a passive experience, this circulation sequence is much more suggestive and imaginative, because in this you are *expecting* to experience specific sensations. So either you will subtly feel *or* you may gently imagine the sensations described below.

As in the first couple of MAP practices, you may have someone read the following outline while you lie with your eyes closed. But thereafter, direct your attention to the CAT sequence directly following the MAP sequence, quietly on your own.

Phase 1

Now, as you finish the MAP, continue focusing for a moment on the top head surfaces—the scalp, temples and brow. No matter how relaxed you may already feel throughout your body's muscles, imagine that there is a little bit of residual tension in these surface head muscles. Now imagine that each time you feel yourself exhaling, those little bits of remaining tension are gently draining away. It's as if the entire upper surface of your head is made of molasses, and every time you feel your breath leave you, you also feel the molasses soften and melt and gradually flow down off the top of the head, and down through the brow and temples, and down along the sides of the head.

Now, during the next several exhales, imagine the insides of your eyes getting softer and softer, slowly dissolving and draining away, down through the inside of your head.

Next, be conscious of your cheeks softening with each exhale, and slowly melting down into your jaw muscles, which are also gradually softening and melting.

Overall, the last slightest bits of residual tension are draining out of your upper head surfaces and facial features, and are flowing down through the softening, loosening neck . . . leaving your head feeling drained, slack, empty, blank, expressionless, lifeless.

Phase 2

Now imagine that all the tension and pressure that have been draining out of the head and face are flowing from the neck and down deep into the right and left shoulders. But as they flow into the shoulders, they feel as if they are transforming into a sort of soft, melted warmth. Very gradually, with each exhale, the shoulders feel warmer and warmer inside.

Imagine that the insides of your shoulders are like pools or reservoirs, and a gentle, soft fluid warmth is slowly filling them up. Continue to feel, or imagine how it would feel, if your shoulders slowly filled completely with soft, radiating warmth.

Phase 3

Now, with each exhale, as all tension drains out of the head and face, as warmth continues to flow deep into the shoulders, the warmth begins to overflow from the shoulders down into the upper arms, both left and right. At first, you feel, or imagine feeling, as if the warmth gently seeps down through the deep inside of the upper arms, and then begins to spread and radiate outward to the skin surfaces.

Now, with each exhale, more warmth releases from the shoulders, like gentle waves of melting sensation, spreading farther down through the arms and forearms, gradually flushing out toward the skin surfaces; finally moving through the wrists into the deepest flesh of the hands, and even spreading slowly into the fingers down to their tips.

Now become aware of your whole body again. You can feel the combined effects of the muscle and circulation routines (MAP + CAT)—vaguely heavy arms and legs; your back sunk into the surface you're lying upon; your breathing rising and falling easily; your head and face muscles feeling drained and empty, blank and expressionless; your shoulders, arms and hands feeling deeply warm and heavy.

Now leave everything just the way it is, remain totally unchanged and passive, and open your eyes—ending your self-awareness practice routine as usual.

EAR
(EXHALE-AIDED RELEASES)

This technique is the first step in translating your relaxation skills from a formal routine, practiced in private, into a skill you can use in various ordinary real-life circumstances. In just ten to fifteen seconds, this releasing technique (EAR) helps you experience the qualities of muscle slackness and bodily calm you have enjoyed during the full practice routines (CAP + CAT)—not as deeply, of course, but sufficiently for all your unconscious physical tension to drain away momentarily.

Do this EAR technique every time it comes to mind. Don't pause to figure out if you have time enough, or to plan the details of it, or get yourself ready. It's much simpler than all that. If it occurs to you, just go right into it.

You may be surprised how often you can pause and physically release youself, without interfering with your normal activities or busy schedule—for example, while waiting for an elevator, or for a red traffic light to turn green; or for someone to answer a phone you've just dialed; or for someone to get something to show you from another room, or to get something from the house as you're both leaving home to go out; or while the train you're riding is stopped in a station (where you're not getting off); or while waiting for your car to warm up a bit; or during ads on TV; or between finishing one activity or piece of work and deciding what to do next; or while being bored by a story you've heard before; and so forth.

Literally dozens of times a day, you'll find youself physically free to let go for a moment. All you have to do is get into the habit, and it will pay off. You will be training your mind to monitor your body's unecessary, previously unconscious muscle tension, and get into the habit of letting it go.

At the instant it occurs to you to loosen up, then, here's what you actually do:

0. If at all possible, let your eyes fall closed.
1. Draw a comfortably deep breath, preferably into the deeper end of your lungs (this is diaphragmatic breathing). As you let the breath go, allow your whole body to loosen and go slack at once. Feel your entire musculature relax and soften. As you let go, recall how your body feels at the end of a good, deep, full-practice routine (CAP + CAT), and let your body sink toward

that feeling of slackness and heaviness—all in one long, comfortable exhale. (Don't worry if you're standing or sitting: you will not fall over. If you're standing and want to let your eyes close, you can keep your balance by placing your hand on something solid next to you.)

2. Draw a comfortably deep second breath. As you inhale, randomly choose a particular muscle (or pair) in the head, neck or shoulder area. Usually you'll find yourself focusing on a muscle that you suspect to be tense—the brow, the jaws, the shoulder-lifting muscles. As you exhale, focus all your awareness in that specific muscle, and imagine you feel it dissolving, draining of tension even more completely than it might have during exhale number 1.

3. Draw a comfortably deep third breath. As you release it, focus inside your forearms and hands, and imagine them feeling warmer and heavier, as if you just completed the CAT, except that instead of lying heavily on the floor, they are hanging at your sides or lying in your lap.

4. Open your eyes and continue about your business. No judgments, no analysis. Just let it go at that. You don't have to "perform" this technique—just do it, with your awareness clear and inward for the moment, but without effort. With practice, its value will become more and more obvious.

Now, to deepen the effectiveness of the EAR technique, to relate it more vividly to the deeply relaxed experience of the full-practice technique, try the following:

Each time you have completed your CAP + CAT (full practice) patterns, and are about to open the eyes, wait a moment. Remain in your physically passive, dissolved, floating state, with your eyes closed, and imagine yourself in a typical EAR situation (for example, waiting for a red light, or during a TV ad, etc.). Fantasize the situation just as clearly and completely as possible, then visualize and feel yourself pausing, doing the EAR, and see yourself there in that real-world situation, feeling as deeply relaxed as you actually are (at this end-of-practice moment).

Then fantasize a second real-world situation, and a second three-breath release. Include this fantasy of one or two EARs at the end of every full-practice routine (CAP + CAT) from now on.

This combination of CAP + CAT + fantasized EARs will help train your mind to expect and accept the two experiences simultaneously—that is, relaxed muscles and worldly environments.

Do not do the EAR only when you are aware of being tense. Simply do it every time it occurs to you. We don't want this technique associated only with need. Instead, it should be done independently of time, place or circumstances, and as often as possible. The purpose of the EARs is to develop, eventually, a constant *habit of being relaxed,* a built-in self-monitoring and self-releasing habit in your mind and muscles.

SHOP
(SLEEP HABIT OPTIMIZATION PROCESS)

Good sleep is fundamental to good health. Lack of sleep will hurt you either immediately or eventually.

On a day-to-day basis, pain, stress and anxiety may be disrupting your night's sleep, leaving you fatigued the next day. The fatigue reduces your body's ability to cope with stress and discomfort, so so that you are even more uncomfortable and probably more anxious. This makes it more likely that the following night's sleep will be spoiled. And so you enter into a vicious cycle of stress and pain → anxiety → insomnia → fatigue → increased stress and pain.

Or perhaps you cheat on your required rest, staying up to watch late television, for example, getting less sleep than you should for extended periods. And perhaps your body has apparently adapted to operating on a tired basis. But this will catch up with you in the long run via serious disease or disorder, increasing vulnerability to stress symptoms, and faster aging.

It is possible to normalize or optimize your sleep cycle, even if you are still coping with stress-related symptoms. The secret is to be completely relaxed physically *before* actually falling asleep each night, for a period of several weeks. Meanwhile you've been learning to reduce your tension levels, thereby reducing your symptoms. With better rest, of course, your improvement will be even more dramatic. In addition, being well rested will be of great general benefit to your health and sense of well-being.

The way to become deeply relaxed physically before falling asleep is to follow a very slow, detailed version of the original MAP (Muscle Awareness Pattern). Therefore, each night when you are *completely* ready for bed . . . with nothing left to do except waiting to fall asleep . . . with the lights low or off . . . with no background radio or TV, etc.:

Lie still in bed, flat on your back, as you did on the floor in the original MAP—except you may use your pillow(s) under your head and/or your knees, if you wish. Let your eyes close and begin to focus on how your breathing feels. Be in no hurry to shift your attention to any other parts of your body, even though you may be aware of them (for example, a sense of your arms and legs softening and getting heavier). Continue to let your mind dwell quietly on the feel of your breathing for perhaps several minutes, no matter what else you may also think of, and despite any temporary mental wandering.

When this breathing focus becomes more of a mental effort than a passive meditation, then begin to focus deep inside the centers of your arches. Continue to focus into a physical sense of them for a few moments. Become conscious of the subtlest feelings in your arch muscles. Now shift your focus to an awareness of the physical existence of your toes (without moving them); then your ankles for a moment; then your heels; then back to the centers of your arches.

Then follow this very detailed pattern throughout the rest of your body, focusing first in the familiar muscle centers of the MAP, then becoming conscious of the physical existence of surrounding parts. For example, from the calves, move your focus around to the shins, knees, ankles, and back to the calves . . . from the thighs, around to the backs of your knees, buttocks, pelvis, back to the thighs . . . from the palms, to the fingers, wrists . . . and so forth.

Continue this style until you either fall asleep or complete the entire MAP. If you actually complete the routine in the above fashion (which could take most of an hour if done correctly) and yet you are still mentally awake, then *do not be concerned about not being asleep*, because by this time your body is deeply relaxed. You are getting excellent *physical* rest anyway, and it's usually true that if you're this relaxed and haven't fallen asleep, then your brain apparently doesn't really *need* the sleep at this time. Don't second-guess your own physiology. Instead, in this situation, enjoy yourself: dream, fantasize, speculate, ponder decisions that need making, consider problems that need solving, and so forth. You're relaxed, so don't be afraid to entertain any subject of thought. Many people find this physically calm, mentally clear state very attractive and productive. If you think of something you want to write down, get up and do so. You won't spoil any magical physical state. In fact, upon returning to bed you may fall asleep more readily than ever.

More often than not, however, you will fall asleep long before completing the slow, detailed MAP. In fact, you may wake up the next morning and not remember getting any farther than the legs. If so, then in the following night's pre-sleep MAP, after the breathing focus, begin the muscle awareness with the palms, forearms, etc. On another night, begin the MAP from the scalp/temples/brow, and proceed downward in reverse sequence, with surrounding details, of course, as described above. In other words, vary your starting point and direction of sequence, so that over a period of weeks, all muscle locations will get some pre-sleep attention, even though you are beginning to fall asleep more and more quickly with continued use of this technique.

Therefore, nightly for several weeks, while you're lying waiting to fall asleep, you'll focus on breathing and muscle awareness. Don't be concerned with when and if you actually fall asleep. Remember, you can't control that anyway. And any attention you give to such thoughts, as "Am I asleep yet? No, I'm not, and good grief, it's 3:15 A.M. Boy, am I going to be tired tomorrow!" doesn't help you to fall asleep any sooner, and may help you worry into staying awake longer. So instead of focusing on whether you're asleep yet, or what discomforts you feel, or what house sounds you hear, focus on breathing and muscle awareness each night until you are either asleep or so deeply relaxed physically that it doesn't matter.

Some extra hints about sleeping:

- Never *try* to fall asleep. Sleep isn't *done,* it just happens when your mind and body are ready. The best you can "do" is eliminate the things that may be keeping you awake, such as unconscious muscle tension. If you're both mentally and physically restless and can't get comfortable, don't fight it; get up and do something, anything, for a short while (even though you're not really interested, force yourself). You'll soon feel quite tired. Then return to bed and follow the SHOP outlined above.
- Do the SHOP lying on your back, even though you may be used to falling asleep on your side. Either you'll fall asleep on your back, which is good for you, or you'll turn onto your side as you lose focus and begin to drift off.
- Use pillows in such a way that your neck and head extend straight up from your spine, without twisting or bending sharply.
- Be sure your bedding is firm enough to support your body evenly, especially along the spine, without sagging.
- If you're especially sensitive to small noises while waiting to fall asleep, buy a small, plug-in white-noise generator (in audio or medical supply stores).
- *Do not eat* for at least three to four hours before going to bed. Drink, O.K. Eat, *no.* Eating not only stimulates your metabolism just when it should be slowing down, but it also is a major factor in gaining excess weight.
- Absolutely avoid sleeping pills except in emergencies. They are addictive, and soon become counterproductive.
- If you wake up in the middle of the night, and don't fall back to sleep within ten to fifteen minutes, then simply begin the pre-sleep MAP, or SHOP, as usual.
- Remember, sleep patterns are influenced by many factors, and are hardly ever uniform from one night to the next. But you can *train* your sleep to be more reliable and of better quality. Like any complex habit, sleep is not changed easily or quickly. But like any habit, it *can* be retrained. You must use the pre-sleep MAP, or SHOP, consistently for several weeks, and follow the above

guidelines as nearly as possible. Then you will enjoy gradually better sleep at night and feel more rested and comfortable daily.

POD
(PROCESS OF DESENSITIZATION)

Now you will begin to apply your new relaxation skills to specific situations, in order to change the way you react to the world around you.

First, take a full sheet of paper, sit down for a few minutes, and write out a list of people, places, activities and circumstances that you know produce tension in you. You should include only those items which come up regularly in your life—daily, weekly, etc. For some common examples of stressful items that many patients have included in their lists, consider the following:

- dealing with your spouse
- dealing with an in-law
- dealing with your own parent(s)
- dealing with your own child(ren)
- dealing with any children
- dealing with a certain acquaintance
- dealing with a certain co-worker
- dealing with or just facing your boss
- meeting deadlines
- making an important decision
- giving speeches or oral reports
- taking a test or exam
- making a sale
- competing, at work or games
- driving in heavy traffic
- driving long distances
- driving on parkways, bridges, or through tunnels
- being in an elevator
- being in a crowded room
- being in a very small space

- being in a very wide open space
- looking down from a height
- seeing insects, spiders, mice, etc.
- periodic unexplainable anxiety feelings
- going to bed to sleep
- waking up/getting up in the morning
- initiating sexual activity
- experiencing annoying symptoms such as nausea, dizziness, weakness, chills, etc.
- onset or continuation of pain symptoms
- visiting a doctor
- visiting a dentist
- taking pills
- swallowing food
- playing a particular sport
- cooking, cleaning or other housework
- typing or other desk work
- figuring your tax return
- balancing your checkbook or budget
- reading for extended periods
- any other person, place, activity or situation

Include in your list only those things that cause a distinct physical tension or anxiety response in you. Some may be very strong, some a lot milder in their effects on you. But they all should be things that come up regularly or periodically.

Keep this list with you, and for the next week or so, when you notice yourself tensing up over anything at all, make sure you add that cause to your list.

As soon as your list has at least a half-dozen entries, you can begin the Process of Desensitization, by which you will learn to be at ease with those very things that used to get you tense.

This process is not a matter of being clever or imaginative; it's simple and obvious once you start it. But in order for it to work well for you, you must follow this strategy consistently for at least several weeks without being impatient for dramatic results. Remember, your stress reactions have developed and become ingrained in you over a long period of time. A lot of your physical tension behavior is unconscious and reflexive habit by now. This kind of maladaptive learning is not reversible overnight. As in learning *any* skill—or *un*learning any bad habit—it takes a while to create or undo behavior patterns. And you will do so only by consistent practice.

So your strategy now is to practice being physically relaxed in the face of things that have made you tense in the past. For the first target of your training, look over your list. Choose an item that is moderate in its effect on you (not your strongest tension producer, and not the weakest). Also, if possible, let it be something that comes up pretty often (more than once a week). An additional advantage would be if it's something that occurs at specific, predictable times. This makes it much easier to prepare for, with the appropriate training steps we will discuss below.

Now I'll describe the Process of Desensitization by using an example. You can apply this strategy to your own first target choice.

Let us suppose you work in an office with a number of other people, and each Monday and Thursday at 2 P.M. there are staff meetings at which each individual must give an oral progress report on his or her work. Let's assume you find yourself tenser as each meeting approaches. Maybe your stomach gets tense, or your hands get clammy. Or even worse, you become short of breath, your mouth gets dry, your thinking gets anxious and unclear. Perhaps Monday and Thursday mornings you tend to awake with a dull headache, feeling depressed, and wishing you didn't have to face the day. Perhaps you have little appetite for breakfast or lunch. Maybe your smoking increases as two o'clock draws near.

Yet probably your report is usually O.K., or is only superficially criticized by your cranky and never satisfied supervisor. And there you are, still on the job, not fired. So maybe you've asked yourself, why be so tense about giving your report at each meeting?—which you evidently handle satisfactorily. Are you afraid of the boss's criticism? —your peers' disrespect?—disappointment in yourself?

Well, it doesn't matter what the tension trigger is. You can learn to be at ease in this recurring situation. Here's how:

Step 1

At the end of each full practice routine (CAP + CAT), before opening your eyes, when your body is feeling deeply relaxed, start to clearly fantasize yourself at lunchtime before the next staff meeting. See yourself eating lunch, thinking of the upcoming meeting, yet feeling as completely relaxed as you actually do now (since you're imagining all this while lying still at the end of your practice routine). Then imagine yourself an hour later, at your desk, getting your papers ready for the meeting, maybe feeling some butterflies or tension in the stomach. Your fantasy continues: Someone calls out, "Meeting in twenty minutes," but see yourself breathing a little deeper and remaining muscularly loose, just the way you feel now (in the end of your routine). Next, see yourself getting up to go into the staff meeting, checking your watch . . . walking into the meeting room . . . taking a seat . . . your boss arriving, looking cranky . . . a couple of co-workers who rub you the wrong way come into the meeting room, being their usual obnoxious selves . . . and so forth. And throughout this clearly fantasized scene, imagine yourself remaining aware of your breathing and loose in your muscles, feeling as bodily calm as you do right now (in your practice routine). See yourself remaining in this physical state right up to the moment the boss calls your name for your report . . . continuing to breathe fully and stay muscle-loose through your first several sentences.

Important: You should envision that whole sequence of events as clearly and realistically as possible, seeing and hearing everything you would in the real-world situation. If at any time during the sequence you notice yourself actually reacting to your fantasy— becoming tense, in even the slightest way—then never mind the fantasy for a moment. Instead, focus on the depth of your breathing, be aware of the feel of all your muscles, and let yourself sink back into a completely relaxed state again. When you feel as completely limp and dissolved as you were before, then return to the fantasy and continue it where you left off.

Each time you feel any physical tension at all, let go of the fantasy, focus on letting yourself sink into a completely relaxed, calm state again, deeper with each exhale. Then continue the fantasy until it's complete.

Step 2

Now you're out in the real world. It's lunchtime before the staff meeting. Take a few minutes, alone if possible, sit comfortably, and do some Exhale-Aided Releases (EARs). When you feel nice and slack, play the same fantasy sequence again in your mind, while feeling your muscles remain slack.

Step 3

Do more and more EARs as meeting time approaches. It's just a matter of giving enough extra attention to breathing a little deeper and remaining muscle-loose as your target time approaches.

This strategy is designed to train your body to remain relaxed in those very situations you used to brace yourself for. It may feel "natural" for you to grit your teeth, to become tight-stomached, when you're anxious. But even if something bothers you mentally, emotionally or psychologically, there is nothing to prevent you from learning to let your *body* relax into it and be *physically* comfortable. You can learn to be mentally and emotionally responsible and concerned, without having to suffer physical symptoms. It's only a matter of consistent practice.

The basis of the above strategy is to give you repeated experience with the combination of a tense situation and a relaxed body. At the end of your practice routines, the relaxed body is real and the tense situation is fantasized. Then when you're out in the real situation, you let your mind and body "pretend" you've just finished a practice routine, which leaves you feeling physically loose and calm.

After a week or two you will begin to find that your first target of desensitization (staff meetings in the above example) is causing you less and less tension. Now you should look at your list again, choose another stress-producing subject or situation, and begin to practice the same strategy toward *it*. Meanwhile continue your desensitizing of the first target for as long as it takes until you find that situation simply doesn't "get to you" anymore. Every week or so, begin a new target, while continuing any that are already in training until they become insignificant as problems for you.

You'll probably find that each new target you begin to work on gets easier, quicker to learn to relax into. This is because, besides learning how to stay loose with each new training target, your mind is also learning how to leave your body loose in general—how to be relaxed at will, no matter what the situation. Not only will you learn to deal with specific situations, but you also acquire the general skill of being physically relaxed by habit, by style.

What will have happened is that you will have become more skillful at the Process of Densensitization itself. Your mind and body become quicker at anything they practice regularly, of course, including relaxation in the face of old tension-producing circumstances.

Above all, enjoy yourself. Enjoy watching yourself gradually learning to be calmer. As always, with all these relaxation routines and application techniques, you will do best if you concentrate on the methods themselves and not on any immediate "results." Let yourself be absorbed with the style of the practice patterns and the methodical steps of the application techniques. Then you will find that the results come automatically, of their own accord.

Fortunately, muscular relaxation is not the only way to combat stress. A new science, called applied kinesiology, helps you reduce stress in three ways, rather than one. And as you'll see in the next chapter, you needn't be successful in all three areas to relieve stress-related symptoms.

7

Applied Kinesiology:
The Science of Stress

In the preceding chapters, we have been talking about chronic pain caused by stress rather than by disease or injury. Stress-related pain has proved to be the most difficult to treat because the source is so elusive. A symptom may arise in one area of the body, like the head or stomach, but the cause is a systemic strain. More than you have to treat the individual symptom, you have to relieve the strain.

A new science, applied kinesiology, addresses itself to relieving internal stress. In treating tension-related problems, kinesiologists are strongly emphasizing the role that dental distress, the TMJ Syndrome, plays. According to their studies, jaw imbalances can precipitate 70 percent of the chronic neurological disturbances with which most patients suffer. These problems include muscular pain, circulatory disorders, and sensation disturbance in the arms and legs.

The theory behind applied kinesiology, in the simplest terms, concludes that each of us has a stress threshold. We can endure all kinds of chaos and annoyance until that threshold is approached. After that, even the slightest upset will cause the brain to send out inappropriate messages to the body, called dysponetic signals.

These signals order the body to go on red alert. A mental danger sign flashes. Muscles brace for action. Adrenaline is pumped into the system. Blood rushes into the trunk of the body. You are ready to attack or to flee. Most of the time, however, you have no immediate threat to fight or to run from. The disturbance that

triggered the command for self-protection was aggravating, but
harmless. All the tension in your body has no outlet so it collects in
the system.

The kinds of distress that cause dysponesis have been broken
down into five categories: (1) dental—jaw imbalances, improper
occlusion, poor swallowing habits; (2) dietary—eating refined
sugars and foods loaded with salt, preservative or other chemicals,
the lack of necessary nutrients inherent in most American diets; (3)
environmental—pollution, poor working conditions, high noise
levels, any noxious agent in our surroundings; (4) psychological—
emotional problems such as marital discord and dissatisfaction with
work, or stresses such as work pressure and financial difficulties; (5)
trauma—milestone and unusual life events such as birth, death,
graduation, divorce, illness or injury.

Let's say that the average person has a stress threshold of 100.
This person is in college in a small town. Dietary distress is 25,
dental distress is 40 due to a jaw imbalance, environmental is 10,
psychological is 20, and there is no trauma. This student graduates,
gets a job and moves to a big city. Now dietary distress is 25, dental
is 40, but environmental is 25, psychological is 30, and trauma is
20. The graduate is over the stress threshold by 40 points. Whenever
a sudden noise or movement occurs, this person feels the rush of
adrenaline into the system and is aware, for a moment, of the
quickening heartbeat.

What happens to all the tension being collected in the system?
Even though you aren't conscious of it, the natural balance of your
body is being disturbed by the tension. The muscles aren't able to
return to their proper resting positions. They are continually
contracted and eventually go into spasm. Spastic muscles may press
on blood vessels and interrupt proper circulation. Nerves may be
pinched, causing pain or a lack of feeling in parts of the body.
Smooth muscle of the organs can be affected too, causing them to
function improperly.

These changes in the system manifest themselves as migraine-like
headaches, muscle-contraction headaches, neckaches and backaches, poor circulation in hands, legs and feet, as well as internal

disorders like high blood pressure or ulcers. The body has the capacity to relieve all these disorders. You don't need long-term drug therapy or surgery for the majority of these cases. But the body won't put energy into healing itself until the emergency signal, that dysponetic message, is turned off. While the body is in dysponesis, it will turn as much as 90 percent of its energy toward defending itself, ready for the imminent attack that the brain keeps broadcasting. Only 10 percent of the body's resources will be devoted to keeping the system in proper running order. If you reverse the proportion of energy going into defense with that going into maintenance, the body will begin to restore a healthy balance in the system.

This information is not news to the medical profession. However, the applied kinesiologic steps taken to achieve a healthy equilibrium in the system are news. In the past, most health professionals concentrated on removing the psychological or environmental stressors from a person's life. But these are usually the most difficult components to control. Leaving a job or a community because the environment is disturbing can be as traumatic as staying there. And many psychological stressors are too complicated to remove.

Applied kinesiologists concentrate on relieving distress where the most immediate results will be produced. Dental distress is the easiest to treat and leads to profound results within a day or a week. A jaw imbalance, given the right environment, can lead to the TMJ Syndrome, resulting in symptoms ranging from disturbed circulation to muscle spasms in the head, neck, shoulders and back. It can account for as much as half of the points on your stress threshold scale. Reposition the jaw and your daily stress may fall well below the critical threshold without your changing job or residence. The result: no symptoms.

Another approach, often used in conjunction with TMJ Syndrome treatment, is nutritional guidance. Dietary distress can comprise one third of the points building up to your stress threshold. If you adhere strictly to the new eating regimen, and comply with the supplement prescription, this distress can be eliminated in as little as two weeks.

Diet is an individual matter. What is good for one person won't necessarily benefit another. For a thorough nutritional work-up, you'd have to visit an applied kinesiologist or a nutritionist. However, there are some universal guidelines that many of you can follow to decrease your dietary distress without the aid of a professional:

1. Caffeine is not good for the body. It may give you a kick in the morning, but you'll plummet by ten-thirty.
2. Refined sugars are a poor source of energy. Replace them with carbohydrates found in fruits and other naturally sweet foods.
3. We've accustomed ourselves to eating grossly oversalted foods. Leave the salt shaker off the table, and try using herbs to replace salt in cooking.
4. Processed, precooked, frozen or refined foods don't supply the bulk or the nutrients that we need. Needless to say, they don't give us the richness of flavor that fresh foods have, either. Think about it for a minute: Is it really easier to heat up a frozen salisbury steak dinner than to cook a fillet of sole?
5. The chemicals used to process foods—colorings, preservatives, artificial flavorings—are not always good for the body. Since we have no way to distinguish additives that are good for you from those that are harmful, we generally advise patients to avoid all of them as much as possible.
6. Eat three meals a day unless otherwise directed by your primary-care physician. Dieting is no excuse for abusing the body; neither is oversleeping. You can't expect mind and body to function well if you don't nourish them.

These are the basic dietary rules by which anyone interested in obtaining optimum health and increasing his or her stress threshold should abide. Our next chapter will detail the balanced diet and the use of fresh, unprocessed foods.

After you've made these initial changes in your diet, you can go one step further and receive nutritional guidance for supplementation to your food intake. Many of us have a deficiency of vitamins or minerals which can't be corrected just by altering our eating habits. Complaints such as constipation, gastrointestinal distress and chronic fatigue can result frequently from such deficiencies. Too often they are treated with potentially harmful drugs when a safe supplement regimen would suffice. And of course, a drug will affect only the symptoms, where the supplementation can remove the underlying problem causing the dysfunction. Chapter 9 will go into the kinds of supplements in more detail.

Applied Kinesiological Testing

Perhaps the most remarkable discovery in this science is applied kinesiologic diagnostic testing. Researchers have found that the body will "tell" them what is wrong if it is "asked." Let's look at a sample test.

You have chronic headaches and seek out the help of a medical practitioner with a background in kinesiology. After an oral history is taken, he or she will test you to discover the source of the pain. One test for a jaw imbalance may be included. The practitioner will ask you to put out your arm. He or she will lay one hand on your shoulder and rest two fingers of the other hand on your wrist. You will be instructed to open your mouth and resist the practitioner's attempt to push the arm down. For the sake of this example, let's assume that you were not overpowered. You tested strong.

Next, the practitioner asks you to clench your teeth and resist in the same manner. This time, you find that you have no strength in your arm at all. The practitioner exerts the slightest pressure and the arm goes down. Now you tested weak. This tells the practitioner that at least part of the problem is in the jaw structure.

We aren't sure what causes the weakness when an imbalance is present in the body, but it occurs consistently. Not only structural disorders will be reflected in the muscles, but biochemical upsets will also cause a drop in strength. Researchers believe that any stress visited on a being will be supported by the whole body, thereby weakening it.

In our practice, we've found kinesiologic testing useful in getting information about structural imbalances in the whole body. We also use it to check a patient's current drug and dietary regimen. Many patients are shocked to see how the painkillers and tranquilizers on which they depended could weaken them. Just slip a tablet on the tongue and the arm drops as if it were weighted. We have yet to test a patient who remained strong when narcotic painkillers and prescription tranquilizers were introduced into the body.

In treatment, applied kinesiologic testing can be used to help the practitioner to prescribe treatment accurately and expediently. We employ it to test the appliances used to balance the jaw. The patient will test weak when the oral appliance isn't adjusted properly. As soon as we grind the plate down to the proper height, the patient will immediately test strong when he or she clenches the teeth. We know the jaws are balanced.

We can also use the test to check for sensitivities to aspirin. In some patients, an aspirin substitute will cause no loss of strength while regular aspirin will cause the arm to go limp.

We've used the arm test here to explain how this procedure works. However, applied kinesiologists can use nearly every part of the body for these resistance tests. And by using this extensive network of body language, these specialists can collect vital, accurate information about disease and disorders that health professionals have never been able to acquire. We believe that medical and dental specialists will use applied kinesiologic testing to make more accurate diagnoses and provide better treatment. But that is a futuristic thought. The real, everyday use of these and other more advanced techniques are still restricted today to the applied kinesiologist's office.

Adjustments

The applied kinesiologist's mode of treatment is the adjustment. Often this is combined with nutritional guidance to maintain the muscular integrity created by manipulation.

Applied kinesiologic adjustments are in some ways related to chiropractic manipulations. To drastically oversimplify their effect, we can say that such treatment will release a spastic, or chronically contracted, muscle and allow it to return to its intended resting position.

To understand how such a simple technique could relieve chronic pains and dysfunction, consider a statement made early in this book: Ninety percent of our chronic pain is caused by muscle spasm. And that's just pain. Our whole system consists mainly of different kinds of muscle. Spasms in tissue throughout the body cause circulation problems, hearing disturbance, even vision problems. Releasing these muscles, allowing them to relax to their designated resting positions, is virtually the only method of relieving this kind of disorder.

Applied kinesiologists can work alone or in conjunction with other specialists. We will work with a specialist when a patient comes to us with complicated muscle-spasm disorders throughout the body. Certainly, a rebalanced jaw will prevent muscle from returning to the spastic state, and we can treat the muscles in the head and neck, but a kinesiologist is needed for complications in the upper or lower back, or other bodily symptoms. However, the applied kinesiologists will reciprocate, and on seeing a patient with TMJ Syndrome, which demands dental attention, will refer the patient to a dentist for that part of the treatment. Certainly, the combination of adjustments and balancing the jaw results in a more successful treatment than either of the two alone.

A case of a pure muscular disorder, such as muscle-contraction back pain, may require only the kinesiologist's attention, since no structural imbalance is involved. In treating any muscle-contraction disorder, however, the kinesiologist will increase the stress threshold as a part of therapy. This is approached first dentally and nutritionally. If daily stress is still above the threshold level, biofeedback, hypnosis and other kinds of relaxation training may be used. Many patients have avoided unnecessary surgery through this unique, safe and effective new therapy.

Applied kinesiology, a science still being born, has opened new doors to healing measures we hadn't considered before. In the near future, it will provide new tools for your health care. This chapter was meant to function more as an alert, calling your attention to this valuable new medical tool, than as a definitive discussion.

In the next chapter, we'll explain how nutrition deficiencies can affect chronic pain as well as your total health picture.

Nutrition: The Cornerstone of Good Health

How many times has your physician reviewed your diet? For most of us, the answer is never. When the doctor comes into the examining room, he or she may ask you about recent tension contributing to a headache or stomach ache, or about the length of time that you've had the symptom, but rarely will diet be discussed. Ironically, most medical specialists concur that proper nutrition is one of the first lines of defense against common health problems, at the same time that most medical practitioners virtually ignore dietary indiscretions when treating a patient.

Samuel S. Bursuk, a New York–based nutritionist and consulting health educator, provided us with this discussion of his approach to balanced nutrition.

Dietary Shortcomings in Our Food

You might think that given the overwhelming abundance and variety of foods available to us at most American supermarkets, our country is not likely to have a nutrition problem. After all, many families have pantries stocked with canned fruits, vegetables, juices, pickles, and even canned meats. Food lockers are jammed with a month's supply of frozen international dinners, not to mention frozen fruits, vegetables, meat and fish, which keep for long periods of time. Even out-of-season produce is shipped across the country or the world to our local market. But nutritionists tell us that this noble effort to keep Americans' stomachs content is also robbing their bodies nutritionally.

The manufacturers of canned, frozen, freeze-dried and ultra-pasteurized foods are entrepreneurs rather than nutritionists. Their objectives are to give the public foods that are easy to prepare and to make the shelf life of those foods virtually infinite. Unfortunately, to accomplish this, they must process most of the nutrients and taste out of packaged food. The six elements for which we eat the beans, fish or other food are lost.

Canned foods, for instance, are completely cooked before they are packaged. Since this lengthy boiling at high temperatures takes away most of the food's flavor, the manufacturer adds salt and sugar. Frozen foods also must be boiled for at least two minutes before they can be packaged. By the time you recook them, they've lost almost as much of their food value as canned goods. We're only talking about the simplest of the processed foods now. Once you get into canned dinners or combined frozen food selections, you find preservatives, flavor enhancers and chemical colorings, all of which camouflage the loss of natural characteristics during processing. While many additives are harmless, none of them are good for human consumption, and some are under investigation for harmful effects.

Even fresh produce and meats are subjected to marketing control—pumped with hormones and colorings, and sprayed with pesticides. All this interference in food production to control appearance instead of quality leads to supermarket deception. You buy the products to comply with the government's nutrition guide-lines, but you don't get the vitamins, minerals, enzymes, fats, proteins or carbohydrates inherent in the foods, since these elements have been processed out. Instead, you are left with a diet loaded with salt, sugar and added starch—none of which nourish the human body properly.

Nutrition and Health

Well, what's wrong with sugar, salt and starch? Don't they give you energy? Certainly, your body needs the sugars in fruits—

naturally occurring sugars—just as it needs naturally occurring starches and salts. However, the manufactured versions of these, used to such excess in processing, often are indigestible. The body can't use them to help it function. At the same time, these substitutes can disrupt your biochemical balance.

Sugar draws calcium into the digestive system. Normally, calcium doesn't enter that system, and when it does, any other food being broken down will be only partially digested. You can imagine the problem a rich dessert can create on top of a large dinner.

When used as a quick source of energy, refined sugar will give you an initial rush, but in a very short time you'll feel low and sluggish—a sign the blood sugar level is plummeting. In contrast, the sugar in dried fruits would give you the needed lift without causing the drop in blood sugar later.

The more we feed our bodies improperly, the more we abuse them. The longer we stay on deficient diets of fast, processed foods, the more severe are the biochemical imbalances and metabolic disorders that result. Excessive salt in the diet has been linked with high blood pressure. Some dyes and artificial sweeteners are known to promote cancer. Heavy cholesterol intake contributes to circulatory and heart disorders in many people.

A prevalent nutritional disorder in the American population is an imbalance in the calcium-phosphorus ratio in the body. These minerals nourish the glands that are responsible for assimilation of food—digesting it and utilizing it in the system. When the calcium-phosphorus balance is disrupted due to lack of these minerals in the diet, you develop a kind of nutritional "Catch-22." Since the ratio is off, you're not digesting your meals properly. You're not deriving the benefits from the foods you eat. Let's say that you recognize the calcium-phosphorus deficiency and load your diet with foods containing these foods. You still won't be able to restore the proper ratio, because the original imbalance prevents the body from assimilating the minerals. The imbalance is self-perpetuating.

You would think that such a drastic alteration in the biochemical balance would be perceived easily. But this kind of malnutrition is insidious, the symptoms of its presence gradually worsening over long periods of time. Our patients rarely come in with a specific complaint. You talk with them a few minutes and they start ticking off the most common symptoms of an undernourished, biochemically imbalanced system. "I don't remember the last time I had a good night's sleep." "I feel sluggish all the time, but I guess that's just old age." "My family says that I'm too touchy, sort of nervous all the time. I remember when they used to say that I had nerves of steel and the patience of a saint." "I don't eat anything—honestly, ask my husband—and I gain weight anyway."

Other common complaints are constipation, depression, irritated colon, nervous stomach, allergies, hypoglycemia, and all the common stress disorders, including headache, backache, stiff neck and TMJ Syndrome.

The malnourished body is a perfect target for muscle-tension disorders. The mineral deficiencies in the muscles make them more susceptible to spasms due to stress or overexertion. The stress threshold is unusually low, as is the pain threshold. The muscles have no nourishment to strengthen them and make them resilient. They are traumatized by stress and are unable to withstand the strain without the proper nutrients. As a result, we suffer not only the fatigue and emotional disturbance of malnutrition, but chronic muscle pain as well.

As you can see, the composite picture of a person with disturbed body chemistry closely resembles that of the chronic-pain patient described in Chapter 2. The majority of chronic-pain disorders are in part due to nutritional deficiencies. Along with stress-reducing techniques and structural balancing, you must correct nutritional deficiencies to ensure long-term relief of muscular pain.

We can restore biochemical balance in two ways, depending on the patient. For the mildest imbalances, we can simply adjust the diet to give the body the proper nutrients with which to balance itself. For those patients with severe imbalances, or those who live in climates where local fresh produce is unavailable, we adjust the diet and prescribe supplements. The end result is the same. The body balances itself and the symptoms of malnutrition are relieved. In three weeks to three months, changes in mood, energy and susceptibility to stress are noticeable.

We emphasize that building the body chemistry by changing the diet is not a curative procedure. A body that is not diseased will naturally heal itself—restore equilibrium after stress. We provide a combination of proper exercise, diet and rest to give the system the necessary elements with which to maintain a healthy body. Many times, symptoms like fatigue, sleeplessness, gastrointestinal distress and constipation are relieved with a simple dietary adjustment.

Most of us, however, pile stress and nutritional abuse on top of each other for years, developing disorders like tension backache or ulcers. Once these symptoms are present, you'll need medical intervention as well as nutritional guidance to treat the physical disturbance while restoring the nutritional balance. Unfortunately, many people treat only half of the problem, getting temporary relief for chronic symptom flare-ups. Yet without a balanced diet, the body can't be the self-healing, healthy system it was meant to be.

Guidelines for Proper Nutrition

We've presented a pretty bleak picture of the availability of good foods in this country. Nonetheless, most of us can make a drastic improvement in the daily diet by using the following guidelines.

1. Build your diet around foods that exist naturally for human consumption. Broadly, this means fruits, vegetables, sprouts, whole grains, nuts, eggs, seeds, meat, fish, fowl, milk and cheese that haven't been processed. A balance of these food products provides us with the six necessary nutrients: vitamins, minerals, enzymes, fats, proteins and carbohydrates.

2. Maintain a natural-high-carbohydrate, low-animal-protein diet. We tend to overemphasize the importance of animal protein when fruits and vegetables are a better source of energy and important nutrients. Fruits and vegetables are most valuable when eaten raw in salads or by the piece. Steaming the vegetables until their color is vibrant, while retaining their flavor and crunchiness, is an alternative, equally healthful method of preparation. After steaming your vegetables, you'll realize that overcooked limp greens not only lose their nutritional properties, but also are unappetizing and tasteless.

3. Use foods in their freshest forms. Although convenience foods make up most of the stock in today's marketplace, we suggest that you work your menu around seasonal, fresh foods.

When you shop for fresh produce, try out the local farm markets in your community. Often the quality of the fruits and vegetables in these markets will be better, since they aren't shipped for thousands of miles, picked before they're ripe or damaged from handling.

If you live in a climate where winters are long, your next choice would be the produce shipped in from warmer climates. And in an emergency, frozen products without added salt or sugar can be substituted for the real thing. We do think that it's best to steer clear of all canned foods, since the nutrients for which you eat them are almost entirely processed out and the additives which you try to avoid are almost always present.

One word about convenience foods: There is no canned or frozen food that is easier to prepare than a salad or even a steamed vegetable. Broiling your own fish, meat or poultry often takes as little time as heating any prepackaged main course. Preparation of simple dishes takes as little time as heating up a TV dinner. And the dinner that you prepare will be far better tasting and more nutritious.

4. Build meals around "monofoods," containing only one or two dissimilar foods, or a combination of like ingredients, as a fruit salad. We have found that the body is not capable of digesting complicated conglomerates of different kinds of foods.

Take pizza, for example. If you were to separate the different ingredients and eat them in three or four courses, you wouldn't develop the anticipated heartburn. The pizza itself, with cheese, tomato, sausage, pepper, or whatever else you like, isn't bad for you. The body simply can't work on such a myriad of ingredients thrown into the stomach all at once.

We espouse layering foods rather than combining them. Many cultures other than ours already use this technique. Quite simply, you eat one food at a time—the salad, a steamed vegetable, some form of protein, and a fruit—all served as separate dishes, one course following another. This way of eating allows the stomach to process each course individually and usually prevents indigestion.

With the layering technique, you are not giving up variety. In fact, when you eat food in this uncomplicated form, you can savor the flavors better. You have just as much variety as you do when combining a dozen ingredients, but you can taste each component of the dish. Many of the finest chefs favor simplicity to overwhelming complication in cooking for just this reason.

5. Check package labels. "Natural" has become a buzz word for food manufacturers. They believe that it sells better to today's additive-conscious consumer. But "natural" foods can contain starch, sugar, salt and other ingredients that are not nutritious.

When you buy packaged goods, see if the ingredients include preservatives, colorings or unnecessary flavor enhancers. Bread, for example, is a product that has few of the nutrients today that it had when it was made from whole wheat, leavening, a little salt, and water or milk. Today the flour is bleached, and starches, sugars and other flavorings have been added. Look for products that contain only the necessary ingredients. Breads should have only four or five, at the most. And check the order of the ingredients. If a loaf of whole wheat bread lists whole wheat as the second to last ingredient, and sugar as the second, you'll know that more sugar than whole wheat was used to make the bread. Even a condiment like soy sauce is produced differently from manufacturer to manufacturer. One will contain thickeners or starches, while another is brewed with only water, wheat and soybeans.

Compare labels when you buy packaged goods to find those manufacturers that use only the necessary, natural ingredients. The product will taste better than one with additives and be better for you.

6. Avoid sugar and salt. A herculean task. These taboo items are found in most foods, with brown sugar being popular in health foods. Pick up a container of any food that you think can't possibly have sugar and salt added, and check the label. More often than not, you're in for a surprise. In health food stores, the granolas are usually made with brown or unprocessed sugar, as are the naturally baked cookies and cakes. Americans, far more than any other nationality, have been conditioned to salt and sugar as a substitute

for the natural taste of food. We don't miss the flavor of the bean, the peach or the muffin if enough of these ingredients have been added.

Spices, seasonings and juices can bring to food what salt and sugar actually take out. They can enhance the flavors of meats and produce naturally. The extra effort to make sauces, salad dressings and other condiments at home—without salt and sugar—is quickly rewarded by the new, rich flavors of food. When sweetness is required, use barley sugar, fructose, sweet fruit or date sugar. For saltiness, use Dr. Bronner's Soya Mineral Bouillon or Dr. Bronner's Sea Dulse. Instead of salt on vegetables, try fresh lemon juice. Use seasoning rather than salt on meats, fish or poultry; then serve them with lemon or lime on the side. And don't be deceived by sea salt or other exotic forms of table salt that are sold in specialty food stores. It's all the same.

7. Avoid alcohol consumption. Most alcohol reacts the same way as sugar in the body, drawing calcium into the digestive tract. Alcohol also ferments food that is already in the stomach, which further disrupts digestion. Much like sugar, alcohol moves swiftly into the system, especially if you drink on an empty stomach. You get an immediate alcohol rush, which wears off in a couple of hours, leaving you tired, irritable and slightly hung over. Regardless of what your grandfather told you about the medicinal qualities of brandy or red wine aiding digestion, stick with soda water and lime during cocktail hours or at parties. It's the one popular drink that leaves you clear-headed to enjoy the party and to get to work the next morning.

8. Avoid drinking with meals. Somewhere in our social history, it became fashionable to offer drinks before dinner and unlimited amounts of wine or water with the food as well as cordials afterward. We can down a pint or more of fluid with a meal. All this liquid gorges the intestinal tract and dilutes the enzymes secreted to break down food. So washing down the sandwich with apple juice or having an after-dinner cup of tea actually sets us up for a feeling of bloatedness and indigestion. Instead of the customary round of drinks, offer fruit to start the meal. The vegetables will provide

enough moisture with dinner, and for dessert you can serve melon or a basket of whole fruits. All these fruit and vegetable courses will quench thirst without disrupting the digestive process.

9. Eliminate caffeine from your diet. Like sugar, caffeine is erroneously connected with energy—a quick booster when you're tired. And like sugar, its effects are more deleterious than helpful.

Caffeine is a stimulant. It will put you on edge, a feeling that many people confuse with being alert. When the caffeine level drops off in a couple of hours, you'll have a rebound effect of drowsiness, headache and irritability. Undoubtedly, you'll head to the kitchen or the coffee shop for another cup of coffee or tea, and the cycle will start again.

Caffeine also constricts blood vessels and upsets the stomach. It's a drug, often used in migraine preparations. It's a stimulant. And it is addictive. Ask any heavy coffee consumer who had to quit cold turkey. Headaches, sluggishness and irritability are common until the body clears itself of the drug. Tea is no better than coffee. Even hot chocolate is loaded with caffeine, as are many sodas.

You do have alternatives to staring at an empty, cold cup in the morning. Herb teas have gained popularity recently and can be found in countless combinations, bagged and loose. Fruit teas, strong and slightly bitter, are commonly imported from Switzerland and make a suitable substitution for coffee, given the tea's gustatorial kick. None of these beverages attempts to mimic the taste of coffee. You might try Pero, Bambu or Cafix if you're looking for a taste imitation. And don't forget to rely on fruits to quench your thirst during breakfast. These beverages are good between-meal stomach buffers.

Typical Menus

At the end of this chapter you will find a few recipes for desserts made without sugar. Samuel Bursuk has provided us with a list of preferred foods, foods to avoid, and salad suggestions. You can make up whatever menus you desire, but the samples we're giving here may help you understand layering and balancing meals.

Breakfast

An important meal, breakfast can be as substantial as this one: Start with a whole orange or freshly squeezed orange juice. Then make your own whole-grain cereal with rolled oats, soy granules, bran, millet and/or puffed rice. Combine these ingredients in any way that pleases your palate. If you like sweetness, use date sugar or fresh fruit, such as bananas, peaches or blueberries, to top off the cereal. Add whole milk and dig in. Then you can move on to the egg course, preferably one or two soft-boiled eggs. And then finish up with cottage or ricotta cheese and a rice cake with butter. If this is a little more than you can manage fresh out of bed, pare down the menu to fruit and either cereal, eggs or cheese with rice cakes for an energetic start to the day.

Snack

We don't advocate eating between meals, but if you are starved midway through the morning or afternoon, try one of the fruit-and-nut snacks, some cheese, plain yogurt, rice cakes or dried fruit.

Lunch

Again, we're looking for that high-natural-carbohydrate, low-animal-protein balance. Start out with a big salad and your own dressing or oil and vinegar. Avocado with the salad is good for you. Tuna, salmon, sardines, cottage cheese, chicken or eggs will also balance out the salad course. Then finish off the meal with a half grapefruit or some other favorite fruit.

Dinner

Note how we layer these courses. Try it a few times and see if you don't feel less bloated after dinner. Start with a mixed salad and your own dressing. Next, have a vegetable course of steamed greens or carrots laced with fresh lemon juice. Following that, serve your fish, meat or fowl, and end the meal with a half grapefruit or some other fruit.

As you can see, foods making up this optimum diet are all available in any supermarket. Of course, you can go to a health food store and buy more exotic products like fructose and date sugar, Cafix and Bambu, whole wheat pastry or bread flour, and other specialty items. If you like to bake or create more complicated dishes using salt and sugar substitutes as well as the more exotic seasonings, start haunting the little specialty shops in your area for these ingredients. What they don't have in stock, they will probably be able to order for you. Some of the products may cost a few pennies more, but the extra pennies could save you dollars in future health-care costs.

Exercise

Exercise is a critical companion to good nutrition. The food you take in is assimilated into the system as the body is moved. If you eat all these good, energy-filled foods but spend your days sitting on the bus, at the office desk, at the dinner table and in front of the TV, the nourishment will be stored as fat rather than used for energy.

Exercise can be more important to your health than a proper diet at times. We have found that active people who eat junk foods process the sugars, salts and chemicals faster and with less detriment to the body than do sedentary people. Exercise helps the body throw off negative substances, helps it cleanse and balance itself.

Like vitamins and minerals, physical activity can't be stored in the body. Two sets of tennis on Saturday don't help you assimilate dinner on Wednesday. You need a daily fitness regimen to make optimum use of a good diet—or to lessen the effects of a binge. You don't have to jog ten miles on the track after work every night. Exercise can be as undemanding as a brisk half-hour walk. The kinds of routines available to you are infinite. You can swim for thirty minutes at lunch, run two miles in the morning before work, or take the dog for a longer walk than usual after work. Be inventive. Make the exercise fit your schedule and personality, and you'll find it to be a pleasure rather than a chore.

Supplements

The key to restoring biochemical balance is good foods and a well-organized diet. The fatigue and nervousness due to malnutrition may be relieved by a simple diet and exercise routine. Nonetheless, Americans continue to look for health in a bottle. The latest boom has been in vitamins. It's the fashion to load up the kitchen table with natural vitamins and swallow fistfuls of them as a preventive measure.

Dietary supplements should be used sparingly. A specialist trained in nutrition should be consulted to determine if a dietary deficiency exists and to recommend the proper supplement.

If at all possible, we try to get the body to restore balance using only the diet and exercise. This is the fastest way to reduce stress in the body systems and to boost energy. However, if the balance is so severely disturbed that the patient is suffering numerous complicated symptoms, or if the available food supply isn't nutritionally sound, supplements may be recommended in addition to the diet and fitness program to aid the body in healing itself.

The Nutritionist's Role

The nutritional aspect of health maintenance is all but ignored in American medical schools. Physicians are familiar only with the most severe and rare diseases that result from vitamin and mineral deficiencies. Yet nutritionists have found that a proper diet combined with a fitness program will prevent many common illnesses and diseases.

The dietary specialist's evaluation tool is the bionutritional analysis. Patients write down everything that they eat for seven days, then they fill out a health appraisal questionnaire, the answers to which indicate probable vitamin and mineral deficiencies. The findings from the questionnaire are corroborated by results of a laboratory blood test series that shows the level of basic elements in the system, as well as a hair analysis, which indicates mineral levels. The nutritionist will then recommend a new diet determined by the findings of the tests, and if necessary, a supplement regimen.

You may see a nutritionist once a week for four weeks, until all the tests are completed and the new diet is put into effect. After that, it is up to the individual to comply with the nutritionist's instructions. The patient is the controlling factor. He or she is the only one who can monitor what goes into the mouth and what doesn't.

For proper nutrition to have the best results, it has to be woven into the life style. You can't leave the diet at home when you go on vacation or to a party. When properly nourished consistently, the body is self-healing, self-balancing, self-cleansing and self-dependent. You don't have to eat fancy or exotic foods. You don't have to memorize complicated diets. However, you do have to discipline yourself to make the sensible choice when faced with a decision between, say, a bowl of fruit and a hot-fudge sundae. The sundae may taste sweet and chocolaty, but an hour or so after eating it, you will feel low and irritable. The fruit will give you energy and keep you going until the next meal.

Nutrition and exercise are two of the most important elements in maintaining good health. They are also the two components of health care over which each individual has absolute control. You determine what you eat and how often you exercise. With a little determination and discipline, good eating habits and a fitness program can be your most powerful weapons against medical problems.

Certainly imbalances in the body chemistry can contribute to chronic pain and other stress disorders, but skeletal abnormalities can often be just as detrimental. In our next chapter, we'll explore osteopathy and how this science of structural integrity relates to your health.

Foods You Should Eat

1. All meats (except franks, salami, bologna, bacon, liverwurst), fowl, fish and shellfish
2. Dairy products, including eggs, butter and cheese
3. All green and yellow vegetables: broccoli, asparagus, celery, cucumbers, artichokes, chicory, chives, endive, escarole, fennel, lettuce, green pepper, parsley, spinach, radishes, watercress, chard, cauliflower, eggplant, cabbage, kale, leeks, string beans, mustard greens, rhubarb: also, olives, dill pickles, mushrooms, herbs, etc.
4. Potatoes or brown rice
5. Fresh fruits such as oranges, lemons, grapefruits, apples, bananas, melons, peaches, pears, watermelons, pineapples, avocados, etc.
6. Green spinach, egg or whole wheat pasta
7. Nuts and dried fruits for snacks
8. Herb tea, Bambu, Cafix or other coffee substitute
9. Cold-pressed vegetable oil, such as safflower, corn and soy oil
10. Apple cider vinegar

Foods to Avoid

1. Sugars
2. White flour and foods containing it
3. Mayonnaise
4. Candies, gum, cookies, all junk foods
5. Soft drinks
6. Coffee
7. Alcoholic beverages
8. Marketed diet foods
9. Salt

How to Make a Great Salad

Ingredients

Lettuce (Boston, romaine, iceberg, etc.), other green leafy vegetables, green pepper, cucumber, radishes, cabbage, celery, chicory, endive, parsley, escarole, artichoke, olives, avocado

Salad dressing

Mix two parts vegetable oil, one part lemon juice or cider vinegar, crushed garlic, and some seasoning such as basil or tarragon, if desired. You may want to alter the ratio of oil to vinegar to suit your taste.

Nutritious Desserts

The craving for sugar is not an easy one to overcome. One way to ease out of the sweets habit is to substitute less harmful sweeteners for sugar in recipes. Joanie Huggins, a nutritionist in Colorado Springs, has put together an entire cookbook of sinfully caloric foods that don't require any sugar, white flour, additives, or preservatives. Her book, *Out of the Sugar Rut,* was published by HAH Publications, Box 2589, Colorado Springs, CO 80906. We're reprinting a couple of our favorite desserts here for you to try.

PUMPKIN COOKIES

½ cup butter	½ teas. salt
¾ cup honey	2 teas. nutmeg
2 eggs	3 teas. cinnamon
1 cup canned pumpkin	½ cup chopped walnuts
2 teas. vanilla	3 teas. allspice
2 cups whole wheat flour	2 teas. orange rind
2 teas. baking powder	1 cup chocolate pieces, or raisins
1 teas. baking soda	½ cup unsweetened applesauce

Cream butter and honey together. Beat in eggs, pumpkin, vanilla, orange rind and applesauce. Mix and sift flour, baking powder, baking soda, salt, nutmeg, cinnamon and allspice. Add to creamed mixture. Mix well. Add walnuts and chocolate pieces, or raisins. Mix thoroughly.

Drop by teaspoons onto well-greased cookie sheets. Bake at 350° for 15 minutes or until lightly browned. Remove from cookie sheets while still warm. Cool on racks. Makes about 4 dozen cookies.

WALNUT JUMBOS

1 cup sifted whole wheat flour   *½ cup honey*
¾ teas. salt   *2 large eggs*
1 teas. baking powder   *⅓ cup molasses*
½ teas. soda   *2 cups oats*
1 teas. ground cinnamon   *1 cup chopped walnuts*
1 teas. ground ginger   *½ cup unsweetened applesauce*
½ cup butter, softened

Preheat oven to 350°. Grease cookie sheets. Sift flour with the salt, baking powder, soda and spices. In large bowl with electric mixer, beat butter, honey, applesauce and eggs together. Blend in molasses, then flour mixture and oats. Stir in walnuts. Drop by spoonfuls onto greased baking sheets, allowing room for spreading, and flatten slightly. Bake above oven center for 13 minutes, until lightly browned. Let stand on sheets about 5 minutes, then use broad spatula to lift onto wire racks to cool. Makes 2½ dozen large cookies.

ORANGE DATE NUT CAKE

¾ cup butter, softened   *¾ cup buttermilk*
¾ cup honey   *1½ cup dates, chopped fine*
4 eggs, separated, beaten   *1 cup pecans, chopped*
2½ cups whole wheat pastry flour,   *rind of 2 oranges, grated*
*   sifted*   *2 tbsp. vanilla*
1/ tbsp. soda   *3 tbsp. unsweetened applesauce*

In large bowl, mix butter and honey. Add beaten egg yolks, vanilla and applesauce, and mix well. Add 2 cups of the sifted flour and soda alternately with the buttermilk. Mix. Mix chopped dates with the other ½ cup sifted flour and mix till well coated and separated. Stir in the dates, nuts and grated rind. Mix. Carefully fold in stiffly beaten egg whites. Grease and flour well a tube pan or angel food cake pan. Pour cake batter into pan. Bake at 350° for 1 hour. Serve with freshly whipped cream or lemon sauce below.

Lemon Sauce

⅓ cup honey
4 teas. cornstarch
1 cup hot water
2 egg yolks, beaten

2 teas. grated lemon rind
4 tbsp. lemon juice
3 tbsp. butter

Mix honey and cornstarch in saucepan. Gradually add the hot water and blend until smooth. Cook on high heat, stirring until thick. Reduce heat and cook 5–7 minutes, until clear. Remove from heat. Blend in quickly the beaten egg yolks, to which a little of the hot mixture has been added. Cook 2 minutes. Add the lemon rind, lemon juice and butter. Dribble over cooked cake, above.

NOTE: This cake has a lovely texture, and is better when served cold. Do not try to slice while still warm. It will stay fresh for at least a week if kept in an airtight container in the refrigerator. Also freezes well.

CARROT CAKE

3 cups grated carrots
2 cups whole wheat flour, sifted
½ teas. salt
2½ teas. soda
2 teas. baking powder
3 teas. cinnamon
1 teas. allspice

1 teas. nutmeg
1 cup honey
1⅓ cup oil
½ cup raisins
1 cup chopped nuts
5 eggs, separated

Mix dry ingredients together. Set aside. Mix grated carrots, raisins and nuts together. Set aside. Beat honey and oil together. Add honey and oil mixture to grated carrot mixture. Add dry ingredients to carrot mixture.

Separate eggs and beat yolks until frothy. Mix into cake mixture. Beat egg whites till very stiff. Fold carefully into cake mixture. Turn into angel food cake pan (tube pan) or 2 loaf pans. Bake for 1 hour at 350°, or until toothpick comes out clean. Cool before cutting.

Topping
8 oz. package cream cheese   1 teas. vanilla extract
juice of ½ lemon   ¼ – ½ cup honey

Mix thoroughly together and spread on cooled carrot cake.

NOTE: This is a very tasty dessert, one of my family's favorites. For a change, try a frosting made from pineapple cheese (available in cheese shops) and nuts. To remove cake from pan, carefully run a knife or metal spatula, using an up and down motion, around edge of cake and around tube, to loosen cake. If tube pan does not have a lift-out bottom, hit pan sharply on kitchen deck, then invert pan and turn out cake.

APPLE CRISP

4 cups sliced apples   ½ cup honey
1 tbsp. lemon juice   1 tsp. cinnamon
1 ¼ cups rolled oats   ¼ cup butter

Put apples in a shallow pan or baking dish. Sprinkle with lemon juice. Combine remaining ingredients and mix to a crumbly consistency; sprinkle crumb mix over apples. Bake at 375° for 30 minutes or until apples are tender.

9

Cranial Osteopathy: A New Look at the Head

For centuries, physicians believed that the bones of the head were immovable. In the early 1900s, a young osteopathic physician named William Garner Sutherland discovered that these bones were definitely, though slightly, mobile in the living body, becoming rigid after death. His work showed us that a strain in the relationship between the skull bones, causing them to become immobile, can affect the whole body adversely. But before we go into the role of cranial osteopathy in a pain-relief program, let's take a quick look at osteopathic medicine.

Osteopathy—the Holistic Medical Science

Osteopaths believe that the body has the ability to sustain health, even to heal itself of minor biochemical imbalances and chronic pain, if its structural integrity is maintained. They have found that most chronic disorders not caused by disease are connected to some part of the body's being improperly positioned, thereby straining not only itself but the organs surrounding it.

For instance, a short leg will stress muscles in the back, neck and head, often causing pain. The osteopath uses a shoe wedge to equalize the leg and relieve the strain caused by the disproportion. This wedge, along with manual manipulation to ease the structural duress, will help the muscles return to their normal resting posi-

191

tions, where they no longer will cause pain. This, of course, is one simplified example of the osteopath's endeavors to maintain the complex structural balance in the human body.

Cranial Osteopathy

This specialty in osteopathic medicine revolves around Dr. Sutherland's discovery of the primary respiratory mechanism. This mechanism functions for the tissues of the head and spine in much the same way that the lungs function for the whole body. The cerebrospinal fluid, which bathes and nourishes the brain and spinal column, circulates in that area about ten to fourteen times a minute, producing a discernible pulse. The fluid reoxygenates the tissues, keeping them vital and functional.

It was this pulsing cerebrospinal fluid that helped Dr. Sutherland understand the purpose of the skull bones' ability to fluctuate. Restriction of this slight mobility would hinder the circulation of the fluid, causing some areas of the brain to receive insufficient nourishment, and consequently to function less than optimally. Also, the compressed skull bones press on sensitive cranial nerves that affect the whole body. Depending on the nerve affected, you could experience hearing or vision impairment, or muscle spasms in the muscles of the neck, back and head, causing pain, dizziness, sinus problems, respiratory disorders, even gastrointestinal distress.

Although the skull is the site where the intracranial strains occur, the back can play a large role in causing the problem. Poor posture, for instance, can stress the muscles and ligaments of the neck and head as well as interrupt the flow of the cerebrospinal fluid into the head. The pull of the muscles and ligaments connecting the head to the spine could freeze part of the primary respiratory mechanism. In this case, the back problem would be an integral part of treating the disruption of the cranial respiratory system.

Osteopaths believe that for most cases of chronic head, neck and back pain caused by muscle spasm, an obstruction of the flow of the cerebrospinal fluid and restricted movement of the skull bones are partially to blame.

Strains on the Skull Bones

Most of us think of our skulls as armor. A bump on the car door or a smack on the back of the head will hurt a little, but it won't do any permanent damage. Cranial osteopaths don't agree. True, a minor bump won't crack the skull, but it might upset this delicate respiratory mechanism that is so central to your health.

Many mild and severe traumas can affect the mobility of the cranial bones. The earliest disturbances can occur while the head is being forced through the birth canal. Osteopaths believe structural abnormalities that develop during birth can account for major defects in the child, including emotional distrubances which mimic mental retardation and hyperactivity. Advocates of this theory feel that a cranial osteopath should be present at the birth of a child to examine the head and release any strains in the relationships of the cranial bones.

In other infants, the slight compression of the skull bones won't demonstrate any symptoms until it is aggravated by bumps and falls in early childhood. Also, certain habits will adversely affect the symmetry of the child's skull over a period of time. Thumb sucking and sleeping with the head turned to the same side every night can traumatize the primary respiratory mechanism. Improper chewing and swallowing behavior is detrimental as well.

If we advance through childhood without any of these bad habits, we're almost certain to pick up a few of the countless adult behaviors that insult the cranial bone symmetry. To name a few, you might wear a bathing cap or winter hat that is too tight; maybe you lug a heavy briefcase or pocketbook in the same hand every day; you might grind your teeth unwittingly, sit at the desk with your head propped up on one hand, or sling the telephone between your ear and shoulder. Other sources of trauma would be exaggerated yawns, long dental sessions, and of course, blows to the head.

If you think you've read this list of accidents and inappropriate responses before, you have. They apply also to the TMJ Syndrome, discussed in an earlier chapter. After all, the jaw is a part of the skull. It also happens to be an easy mark for injury. Any imbalance in the jaw will affect the primary respiratory mechanism negatively.

Osteopathic Treatment

An examination by an osteopathic physician can differ substantially from that given by a general practitioner. The osteopath will be looking for structural integrity and balance in the whole body rather than concentrating on individual symptoms. He or she will press and poke and bend your body until the source or sources of your discomfort are discovered.

Although the cranial osteopath specializes in problems with the skull bones, he or she will do a full body examination, checking for imbalances in other areas that may be affecting the head. Any strains in the primary respiratory mechanism will be released with delicate head adjustments. The osteopath will then treat the rest of the body, restoring balance to the structures supporting the head.

Aside from these manual adjustments, the osteopath will discuss posture and behavioral problems that increase the risk of further intracranial strains and concomitant complaints. He or she may advise carrying a smaller, lighter handbag or briefcase. Maybe new positions for working, reading or studying will be suggested. Exercises to break the teeth-grinding or clenching habit will be discussed. The osteopath might feel that you should wear a different style of swim cap, snorkel mask, ski goggles or sunglasses. Whatever inappropriate habits of yours are contributing to imbalances in the body will be reviewed and altered. If your examination indicates a TMJ problem or other structural abnormality requiring a specialist's attention, your osteopathic physician will refer you to the proper medical professional to treat the disorder.

If your pain is due to some structural imbalance, like a strain in the skull-bone relationships, a curved spine, or jaw imbalance, an osteopath will be able to alleviate much of your discomfort by relieving the internal stresses that cause muscle tension, muscle spasms and subsequent pain. As you learn proper posture and swallowing habits, the stability of the osteopathic adjustments will increase until the structural integrity of your body is sustained in your daily life style.

Our next chapter will discuss another kind of imbalance in the system—hormonal imbalance. This, too, can be critical to the lasting relief of chronic muscular pain.

10

Hormonal Balance and Muscular Pain

When you go to a pain specialist, you may find a series of ten or so questions on the medical history that seem to have nothing to do with your pain: Are your hands and feet always cold? Do you have any trouble with your period? Are you always tired? Are your nails and hair brittle?

These questions may seem to be irrelevant, but they're actually giving the physician the first clues to an existing hormonal imbalance.

Dr. Lila Wallis, an associate professor of clinical medicine at Cornell University Medical College at New York Hospital–Cornell Medical Center in New York City, sees many patients whose endocrine imbalances contribute to a chronic pain. Her ideas about the most common imbalance associated with pain are discussed in this chapter.

What Endocrine Glands Do

Endocrine glands produce hormones and secrete them into the bloodstream. Since the blood bathes every organ in the body, every organ is affected by the endocrine system. An overabundance or a shortage of a hormone frequently has repercussions throughout the body.

How does the hormonal balance affect you, the pain sufferer? A deficiency in some of the hormones makes muscles more susceptible to spasm and subsequent pain. In particular, shortage of the thyroid hormone has been linked with painful muscle spasm. Hypothyroid patients may suffer from any of a number of pains: cramps in the legs and feet; aching back; and most prominently, stiff, aching necks with an associated head pain.

Frequently these patients have done all kinds of exercises and taken muscles relaxants by the bottle. Sometimes the pain lets up for a few weeks, but it always returns. And it always will until the hormonal imbalance is corrected.

How the Muscles Go into Spasm

Of course, muscle spasms can begin in a violent way, such as in a car accident. However, the most common predisposing factors are tension, poor posture, cramped working positions, repetitious movements and sedentary life styles.

For instance, a minor trauma to the neck (exposure to a cold draft, sitting watching TV in a cramped, twisted position, changing light bulbs on a ceiling fixture, washing the ceiling, etc.) may initiate mild discomfort in the neck. The patient unconsciously assumes a slightly hunched posture, to avoid the seemingly greater discomfort of straightening out the neck. As the days go on, the patient freezes in this unnatural bent-over position; a round-shouldered stoop becomes associated with a strained, chin-up position of the head as the patient tries to see objects at eyeball level. This puts further strain on the back muscles of the neck, on the trapezius muscles supporting the head and neck, and on the muscles of the shoulder girdle. Constant contraction of these muscles provokes a painful spasm.

When such a patient hobbles into the office, the first aim is to terminate the painful spasm by straightening up the shoulders and the neck, and bringing the head into a neutral position. Finally, the muscles are able to relax. All the time the patient was stooping to take stress off the painful muscles, he or she was actually putting more stress on them by forcing the muscles to hold the body in one stiff, unusual position. The muscle spasms spread from the neck to the shoulders and back, creating an ever increasing amount of pain.

Thyroid hormone insufficiency predisposes a person to painful muscle spasms and magnifies their consequences. In a patient with a balanced endocrine system, the pulled or strained muscles would be able to relax if stretched and rested properly. In a person with insufficient thyroid, the muscles tend to go into spasm more easily, and stay tight and painful even while treated by a physical therapist. Until the hormone level is restored, the spasms will continue to recur regardless of the physical therapy treatments.

In a woman, a decreased level of estrogen is another predisposing factor to muscle spasm which must be treated.

With the recent unwarranted estrogen-cancerophobia, many postmenopausal women whose back pains had long vanished on physical therapy and estrogen administration stopped their estrogen therapy. After many years of pain-free existence, these individuals once again experienced recurrence of the long-forgotten pains.

The Endocrinologist's Role

Chronic muscle spasms are one clue to a hormonal imbalance, but the endocrinologist will certainly need more exact information to diagnose a problem. Laboratory tests will be required to determine if one or more suspected imbalances exist. The kind of test used depends on the imbalance being studied. And in spite of the numerous tests being used for the diagnosis of hypothyroidism, often its diagnosis can best be proved by means of a therapeutic trial with thyroid hormone.

Of course, we can't write down a standard treatment plan here because each of our patients presents a different problem which needs individualized care. However, some common approaches are used for all our patients.

Our primary concern is to be certain that all the glands in the system are working well. Multiple imbalances are not uncommon. When we've identified the insufficiency or overabundance of a hormone, we use medication to correct the imbalance. In the case of thyroid insufficiency, we prescribe replacement with thyroid hormone.

Rebalancing the system is only part of the treatment, however. To rectify damage already done to the body by the hormone imbalance, we frequently refer the patient to physical therapy. This phase of treatment would be directed at breaking up the spasm by injecting the trigger points, at restoring the muscle tone by limbering tight muscles, and at changing poor posture and behavior patterns that led to muscle stiffness in the first place. One rule of thumb endocrinologist Wallis gives such patients is: Never sit still. Change positions frequently to keep the muscles from freezing and tensing. A simple shift in position every few minutes—such as recrossing the legs, pushing the chair closer to or farther from the desk, stretching backward if you're bending over, or forward if you're leaning back—is very beneficial.

How Safe Is Thyroid Replacement Therapy?

Recently, the popular press devoted a lot of space to stories concerning the risk of breast and uterine cancer's increasing with the use of thyroid replacement therapy. That rumor was based on an inadequate study which led to erroneous conclusions. As a matter of fact, thyroid deficiency has been linked positively with increased incidence of breast cancer. In many controlled laboratory studies, the restoration of the proper level of thyroid hormone, using synthetic hormones, reduced the incidence of breast cancer substantially.

Excessive amounts of thyroid hormone can be associated with cardiac symptoms such as irregular or accelerated heartbeat. Since the amount of thyroid required by a patient may change over the years, every patient must be closely monitored to make sure that he or she is receiving an adequate but not excessive dose. When monitored properly, thyroid replacement therapy is safe and effective.

Treatment by an endocrinologist and by a physical rehabilitation expert need not be sequential, but may proceed concurrently. The physical rehabilitation will be most effective when the hormonal milieu is optimal. A simultaneous approach to chronic pain may save a lot of time and discomfort. Our next chapter will discuss the physical balancing of the body and how these procedures can help you.

11

Physical Therapy: Restoring Function

Physical therapy has long been underrated as a treatment for chronic pain. As the therapists point out, pain is a distress call. And as we've noted throughout the chapters on head, neck and back pain, most chronic pain is connected to a structural imbalance.

The physical therapist specializes in restoring equilibrium in the musculoskeletal system. He or she examines every moving part of the body to ensure that all of them bend, rotate and straighten properly. If an abnormality is found, the therapist's goal is to restore proper position and function of joints and relieve muscle strain, thereby relieving discomfort. If the body is not injured or diseased, this restoration of equilibrium renders the musculoskeletal system pain-free.

Mariano Rocabado, a physical therapist specializing in orthopedic physical therapy, director of the head, neck and facial pain clinic in West Paces Ferry, Atlanta, Georgia, and professor at the School of Dentistry in the University of Chile at Santiago, gave us his impressions of how physical therapy fits into pain control and what you can expect from a visit to a therapist.

What Is Function?

Function is how your body moves, whether you're swallowing, combing your hair or scratching your back. In our bodies, proper function can depend on more than one body part. Here's an example. Hold your arm out in front of you. Notice that the hand doesn't stretch out straight from the wrist. It deviates to one side. Therefore, you will not be able to have full function or extension of your elbow unless you can deviate the hand to one side at the same time. This is an example of biomechanical function depending on two movements.

Many of our simple and complicated functions require two or more body parts to move simultaneously, making the structures that perform these functions interdependent. This is an important factor in treating pain because the ramifications of a dysfunction in one part of the body will appear wherever that part plays a role in function.

Let's say that you have a stiff joint. All the tissues surrounding and interacting with that joint will be affected. One example of this would be the jaw-joint imbalance that we discussed in chapter 3. The imbalanced joint will cause the jaw to alter its normal range of motion as well as its normal resting position. To counter this, the head will change its resting position on the neck and shoulders, and the vertebrae in the neck and upper back will change their relationship to one another in order to accommodate the new position of the head. Finally, the muscles surrounding the jaw and supporting the head will have to change their normal patterns of activity to allow for the shifting in the bony structure.

All these stresses come from the imbalance of the jaw joint. You can see how an abnormality in one place can send shock waves to distant parts of the body.

Structural Balance and Pain

We've talked about structural balance in relation to pain throughout the preceding chapters, but let's look at it in the light of function.

The muscles, ligaments and other tissues that support and move the skeleton have definite, memorized patterns through the central nervous system. They stretch only a certain distance in a predetermined direction, and they return to a fixed resting position. When used in the proper capacity, they remain healthy and pain-free. However, any structural imbalance will demand a change in the soft tissues' pattern of activity. Suddenly the normal resting position is unattainable. The tissues strain. They are continuously tensed and soon become painful.

You might better understand the problem with changing the soft tissues' pattern of activity given this example: Most of us accustom ourselves to working positions that are dependent on chairs and desks, counters or other stationary surfaces. If you've been sitting on one chair in a certain relationship to your desk for five years, and your company supplies a new chair, you may develop back and neck pains. The discomfort will not be due to tension so much as it will reflect the changes in your posture forced by the new chair. After five years, you're asking the body to hold you at a new height over the desk, to position you differently when you're writing, or perhaps to compensate for a greater distance between your desk and the new chair. All these changes in normal function will overload the muscles and joints of your body.

Most muscular pain comes from old, bad habits rather than from new behavior. Inappropriate postures are used for long periods, day after day, year after year. The insult to the body accumulates slowly. Often the pain starts so long after the aggravating behavior was initiated that you forget which habit is the cause of the discomfort.

We find that most chronic pain is caused by minor repeated traumas to the body—in other words, bad habits. Sure we have our share of automobile accidents and sports injuries, but the majority of people we see will tell you that their pain appeared out of the blue. They woke up with it one day. It started suddenly when they reached for the salt or the morning paper.

We know, however, that the pain just doesn't happen. One patient may have held on to a subway strap once too often. Another may have lugged around a heavy briefcase or handbag in the same hand every day. Sometimes what does it is cupping the phone to the ear with the shoulder habitually, or reaching for a tool with the same hand. After months of abuse, the muscles and joints finally give in under the strain. You might feel the pain for the first time, but your body's been in trouble for months—maybe years.

Any repetitive movement for which you don't compensate with some kind of countermovement—like alternating hands when reaching for or carrying something—will cause stiffness and eventual spasm in a muscle. You can compare the body to a car engine. If you run a motor at the same speed all the time, that engine will wear in the same spot every time you use it. The breakdown of the engine will occur much faster than if the motor were run at different speeds, distributing the work load to the whole machine. Similarly, if you give each muscle group periodic rests or occasions to stretch, it will be able to withstand more than the muscle group used every day for the same job.

Where the Pain Comes From

Many misconceptions exist about what causes head, neck and back pain. We'd like to go over the dysfunctions often unrecognized by other medical professionals that the physical therapist routinely treats.

We believe that many chronic pain syndromes start as a result of abnormal joint biomechanics. Joints are innervated, thus they and the surrounding tissues may cause pain. This is true of any joint, be it an elbow, a jaw joint or a neck vertebra. Yet most specialists don't concern themselves with proper function—making sure that the joints are positioned and moving properly—and discomfort persists in joints that are not functioning optimally.

Secondly, we have found that many specialists are looking at only half of the problem. We are balanced creatures. Each of our muscle groups has a reciprocal group with which it interacts. When one of theses groups is stiff or painful, chances are good that the other is suffering too. Often only one part of the traumatized area actually causes pain, and standard medical procedure calls for that one part only to be treated. Unfortunately, the pain won't be permanently relieved until both muscle groups are normalized.

Here's an example. The muscles and ligaments in the front of the neck are rarely examined during diagnosis of head and neck pain, yet these supportive structures are often more traumatized and more in need of treatment than the stronger muscles in the back of the neck.

In many whiplash cases, we find that the specialist notes the trauma in the back of the neck, prescribes a cervical collar to ease the strain on those muscles and to relieve the compression of the neck joints, and sends the patient home. The doctor never looked at the muscles in the front of the neck. Yet the head was thrown not only forward, affecting the back of the neck, but backward as well, wrenching the muscles in the front of the neck. Year after year, the weaker, more traumatized muscles in the front of the neck cause ever more disabling pain because they never healed properly.

This principle applies to all muscle-contraction pain. You have to treat the complementary supportive tissue in any structure to effect lasting relief.

Finally, we have found that the many sensitive structures passing through or near the neck vertebrae are often overlooked as a source of pain. Any posture that compresses the vertebrae in the neck, like looking up for long periods of time or reading with your head bent for hours, can affect the sensitive nerves and vessels in and around the cervical spine. Physical therapists have learned how to evaluate and treat a dysfunction in the neck, as well as how to differentiate pain from disorders it mimics.

What to Expect from a Physical Therapist

The physical therapist is always more interested in where the pain originates rather than where you're feeling it. Sometimes the source and the discomfort are in the same place, but often the source is quite removed from the pain. Therefore, your testimony of suffering will not be as important to the evaluation of your condition as will be the palpation of the joints and soft tissues capable of causing pain.

The first step would be a structural examination. The therapist observes how your body is held—how the head sits on the neck, the relation of the neck to the back, the back to the pelvis, and so on down the body. Next, the therapist will palpate the soft tissues around the joints of the body to check their condition. Then a mobility test will provide information about how the individual joints are moving by themselves and in relation to the rest of your body. These tests give the therapist a clear picture of the structural balances and imbalances in your body.

With the information provided by this evaluation, structural dysfunction that may be causing discomfort can be isolated. In the areas suspected of being in dysfunction, the therapist will examine each joint at every angle to root out the malfunction.

During the examination, the therapist is collecting information not only about muscles and joints, but also about the nerves and blood vessels in the area, and how the state of the joint and soft tissues can affect theses structures, possibly causing present or future symptoms.

Sometimes there are sympathetic and parasympathetic reactions to consider, such as dizziness, nausea, constipation or cold sweat. When the evaluation is complete, the therapist will understand how all your seemingly unconnected chronic symptoms fit together, and how to untangle the physiological dysfunctions in your body to relieve them.

Treatment methods in this field of medicine are mostly physical rather than pharmacological or psychological. The therapist uses joint-liberation techniques to restore the normal function of a joint and to relieve stress on the tissues surrounding it.

If the joint is too painful to tolerate movement, the therapist may use heat or ice treatments to produce relaxation and decrease the sensation in the area. Another form of stimulation used to reduce the sensitivity of an area requiring treatment is the transcutaneous nerve stimulator. This device uses a mild electric current to produce a neural block in the painful joint or muscle. With these pain-reducing methods, a physical therapist can begin treatment sooner without risking the side effects of painkilling drugs.

Aside from the therapist's joint-liberation treatments, you will probably have to retrain yourself in personal habits to keep the joints from going back into dysfunction. You may have to sit differently, swallow with the tongue in a new position, hold your body in a different posture, or change the manner in which you approach other physical activities.

Some therapists use an exercise regimen of thirty minutes a day in which you perform your own exercises or self-mobilization program. We believe that this method doesn't integrate the new behavior into the daily life style, and may lead to overexertion of the muscle or joint in certain zealous patients. Our exercise program runs throughout the day, and requires the patient to do six repeats of a given movement six times a day, the 6×6 method.

Sometimes we connect the exercise with a trigger mechanism, like a sound that the patient hears at work, or a glass left on the kitchen table, or maybe a special ring to remind the patient of some behavioral correction whenever he or she looks at the finger. In this way, you're not just doing an exercise once or twice a day; you are retraining the muscles and joints to work along a new pattern. Developing these new habits is essential so that your progress with the therapist will not be retarded or even repressed.

As with any other therapy, some patients respond faster to treatment than others. Some will feel a complete absence of pain after the first session, while others may take a few weeks to improve. Sometimes the treatments make a muscle or joint sore for a couple of days before it feels better.

The psychological factors in chronic pain play a role in the expediency of the treatment. If you are used to a certain movement hurting, it may take a while to believe that it won't hurt. After a few weeks, though, you observe that you can move without discomfort—not just once in a while, but every time. Finally, you believe that you won't suffer for the newly acquired ease of movement.

Most people with muscular pain—pain not due to disease or defects—can expect to be treated successfully by a physical therapist specializing in orthopedics. After all, once the body is balanced, the muscles can stretch and contract in their normal patterns, and the joints are free to move in the correct manner, there is no reason for muscles to cause pain.

But where are you going to find a physical therapist, no less a specialist in orthopedic therapy? Our next chapter gives you the sources for all the specialists mentioned in this book.

12

Where to Find Help

The medical information presented in this book is not unusually complicated or recently discovered. However, the procedures, examinations and treatment methods are foreign to most illness-oriented, drug-dependent medical practices. If you've suffered with chronic pain for a number of years, you can probably attest to the medical establishment's aversion to physical contact with patients. How many times have the ten or fifteen specialists you've seen touched the place that hurts, prodded the muscles to test for spasms and trigger points, or noted how short one leg was next to the other?

Our approach to relieving pain demands this close attention to the whole patient. And as many of you will discover, your internist or family physician is unfamiliar with this kind of medicine. Many osteopaths, physical therapists, physiatrists and TMJ specialists are familiar with it, however, and these are the professionals that we suggest you call. If you have any symptoms connected with a jaw imbalance, visit a dentist specializing in TMJ for a consultation. If you can't find such a specialist in your area, make an appointment with a cranial osteopath for a diagnosis and treatment as well as a referral to a TMJ specialist if necessary.

Neck- and back-pain sufferers should look into physiatry as an alternative to orthopedics in the treatment of their pain. Always look to the most conservative treatment for pain before submitting unnecessarily to drug therapy or surgery. The physiatrist will help you relieve muscular discomfort, the cause of more than 90 percent of all back and neck pain.

Biofeedback and nutritional guidance are helpful and often necessary adjuncts to relieving chronic pain. Professionals in these fields are rarely included in an appraisal of the chronic-pain patient's symptoms, by standard medical procedure. You have to seek out their assistance yourself.

But where can you find these specialists? In this chapter we're giving you basic guidelines for locating the medical professionals with whom you'd like to consult. These are general instructions. The referrals you receive from these sources will not be recommendations. You will need to evaluate the individual practitioner as you would any other professional whose services you were using.

TMJ Specialists

Your local dental society would be aware of dentists who treat TMJ Syndrome in your area. A dental school in the vicinity also would have a list of TMJ specialists connected with the college. Aside from these local sources, you can write to these two societies for a list of the specialists practicing near your residence:

The American Equilibration Society
211 East Chicago Avenue
Suite 1636
Chicago, Illinois 60611

The American Academy of Craniomandibular Disorders
William Danzig, D.D.S.
2021 Ygnacio Valley Road
Walnut Creek, California 94598

Physiatrists and Physical Therapists

These practitioners are specialists in physical medicine and most often they practice in the departments of physical rehabilitation of medical centers. You will probably be given several names of practitioners if you call the department of physical rehabilitation at your local hospital. You can also contact the following organization for specialized clinics and practitioners dealing primarily with pain:

> Ms. Louisa E. Jones
> Executive Secretary, International Association for the Study of Pain
> Dept. of Anesthesiology RN–10
> University of Washington
> Seattle, Washington 98195

Osteopaths

You'll find a listing for osteopathic physicians in your yellow pages in many locations. Perhaps a better source would be the American Academy of Osteopathy, which can refer you to an osteopath experienced in chronic muscular pain and cranial osteopathy. The local osteopathic society would be familiar with practitioners in your area. If you have trouble finding the local chapter's address, write to the national headquarters at the American Academy of Osteopathy, 2630 Airport Road, Colorado Springs, Colorado 80910, or call them at (303) 632–7164.

Biofeedback Instructors

You can write Francine Butler at the Biofeedback Research Society, 4200 East 9th Avenue, Box C268, Denver, Colorado 80262. She will supply you with a few select names of recommended practitioners in your area.

Nutritionists

We have a wealth of organizations to which you can write for information regarding medical nutritionists in your area. Write to the organization closest to your home:

International Academy of Preventive Medicine
10405 Town & Country Way
Suite 200
Houston, Texas 77024

Academy of Orthomolecular Psychiatry
North Nassau Mental Health Center
1691 Northern Boulevard
Manhasset, New York 11030

International College of Applied Nutrition
P.O. Box 386
La Habra, California 90631

International Academy of Biological Medicine
P.O. Box 31313
Phoenix, Arizona 85046

International Academy of Metabology
1000 East Walnut Street
Suite 247
Pasadena, California 90631

Endocrinologists

Most endocrinologists, like physical therapists, only take on patients referred to them by another medical professional. Our suggestion is that you ask for a referral from a dentist or physician who is knowledgeable in muscle-contraction pain disorders. You want, after all, an endocrinologist who is also familiar with the role of hormones in chronic pain.

13

Patient Histories

We've given you all the facts about chronic muscular pain, and now we'd like to show you the human side of the story. The following are accounts from a few of our patients, whose experiences range from uneventful to life-threatening.

Nancy

I'm twenty-four years old and I've had headaches for five years. They started in my freshman year of college. One day I just got this terrible headache. It really put me out. I lost partial vision in one eye. I even went to the infirmary for a while.

Then it seemed that I had constant headaches. I didn't know why. They were on the right side of my head. My vision was all blurry in one eye too. Well, both my parents have migraines, so I was brought up to think that it was normal to have headaches. And no one told me any different.

I went through the rest of college with constant headaches. I remember waking up every day with this dull thud in my head. It just got worse and worse. And I had a terrific personality change during that time. I got very withdrawn and more and more depressed. I was really antisocial. That didn't make any sense if you considered my past social life.

Just before I left school, I saw several doctors. One of them was my dentist, whom I'd known all my life. He said that I had something wrong with my jaw, but that the pain was mainly in my head. He said, "Well, if you weren't so moody, and if you weren't so anxious all the time, you wouldn't have the pain." I told him that it was the pain that was making me anxious and moody.

Anyway, he wanted to put a bite plate in my mouth, but I wanted to get checked out by some other doctors first. I had brain scans, electroencephalograms, and a whole range of tests for brain tumors and other neurological disorders. One doctor put me on five tranquilizers a day. An orthodontist wanted to put full braces on me. But nobody seemed to know what was wrong with my head. So I decided to go back to my dentist.

This was just before I went to England for three months to work. The dentist and I agreed that the treatment couldn't be successful if I had to leave in a week. So I waited until I got back. My work in England was very physical. I had constant throbbing headaches and terrible backaches. Now I was beginning to believe that I was a mental case.

Finally, I got back and had the plate put in my mouth. It seemed that this dentist was improvising on what he already knew. He kept building up the plate and building it up. It hung down beneath my upper teeth, making it impossible for me to speak or eat when it was in—aside from the discomfort. I'm a performer, so you can imagine what this did for my career.

I got fed up with that contraption and took it out of my mouth. It had helped a bit, but when it was out of my mouth for a couple of days, the headaches, backaches and blurry vision all came back. The dentist said that I would have to wear the plate whenever I had pain. For the rest of my life.

I was bitter and unhappy at that point. I didn't want to talk to friends or go out. I can't imagine how they put up with me. It looked like my life, at twenty-three, was over.

One day I ran into a friend at work. She told me that her sister had been having a problem much like mine and had found a doctor who had helped her. That was Dr. Gelb. I made an appointment that day.

Dr. Gelb put an appliance in my mouth, but on the bottom teeth, where it didn't interfere with talking or eating. It took about six weeks, and then the headaches were gone. And the blurry vision. And the backaches. And the moodiness.

Kathy

For the past twenty-one years, I've been a foster mother. When I started having trouble with my neck, I had five children in the house. That was in 1974. I didn't feel anything in my neck actually. I was having trouble with my hearing and went to an ear specialist. Every time I would visit him, I'd come in with a stiff neck. He tried to tell me that the problem was not just in my ear, but was in the neck too, but I didn't understand him. He spoke with a thick accent. This went on for a while. My neck got worse and worse. Finally, in 1975, I couldn't move at all. One night at two in the morning, I woke up with my chin stuck down to my chest. I was rushed to the hospital, and the orthopedic surgeon said that I needed to be put in traction. So they hooked me up and I screamed, "Oh, my God, my ears." I was in such pain. The doctor said, what's wrong with your ears, and all I could say was that they hurt. The doctor gave me a strong painkiller so that he could keep me in traction.

I went home after a couple of weeks and had to be in traction there too. It was agony. I just sat there and cried all day. And when I tried to do anything, I found that I was terribly dizzy and had a splitting headache.

I got tired of sitting at home and went to see a chiropractor. He said that there was something wrong with my back and he could fix it. Then he gave me some medicine for the dizziness. I saw him every other day for a long time. He was helping, but I went to another doctor to see if maybe the chiropractor had missed something.

I went to this other doctor and he said that I was hyperventilating and that was my problem. That was a neurologist. Then I went to a new internist and he said that the problem was also arthritis in the neck. He gave me some medicine for the arthritis and said that I'd have to learn to live with it.

The next part is almost funny. My husband was in an auto accident and we went to see our family physician. We walked in and he asked me—not my husband: me—what was wrong. I told him that my husband was the sick one and he said that he wanted to examine me anyway because I looked so bad. He noticed that I was avoiding the bright lights. They hurt my eyes. And I was walking like I was drunk because I was so dizzy. This doctor said that he couldn't help me, but he heard of cases like this that were related to a jaw imbalance. And he sent me to Dr. Gelb.

Soon after Dr. Gelb put my bite plate in, I felt better. Now all the neck pain, ear problems, dizziness and headaches are gone. I do have some arthritis in the neck, and that will bother me, you know, in bad weather. But the pain is gone. Like magic. My chiropractor can't believe it.

Sara

I'm sixty-one years old and run a boutique in New York. Several years ago, I had pains in the back of my head. There was also a pulling sensation. Sometimes the pains were so bad that they would wake me up in the middle of the night. I'd be nauseous. Oh, it was the most horrible thing! You can't imagine such pain. And of course, I never could get to sleep. It was just a nightmare. I thought maybe it was a tumor or something.

I saw a neurologist and was told that it was arthritis in my neck. I had to just live with it. Now, this was a prestigious physician. You wouldn't doubt the word of such a specialist. But I couldn't live with it.

I went to several doctors and none of them could help. I also noticed that when I had my teeth fixed, all the problems would get worse. My throat would get so sore. And the muscles on the sides and in front and back of the neck were aching so. The dentist tried to help. He would grind down my teeth. Then once I was in such pain after a visit to his office, I came in crying the next day and begged him to help me. He said he'd try and put this clumsy type of brace in my mouth. He wanted me to wear it all the time. But I speak to people all day long. I couldn't have this strange contraption in my mouth.

This went on for a year. Neurologists gave me painkillers and took x-rays of my head. No one could figure out how to make me better. It took five years from the start of the pain for my dentist to suggest that I see Dr. Gelb.

Finally, I did see Dr. Gelb. He explained what he would do and said he could help me. I was supposed to go on vacation in just a few days, so when he said he'd schedule me in when I got back, I asked if there wasn't anything he could do right then. And do you know that he had a technician make up this rubber mouth guard in a few minutes. He put it in my mouth and the pain—after all those years—started melting away. I could feel the muscles relaxing.

Well, that was the best trip of my life. I can't begin to tell you what it means to sleep for a full night without being awakened by this awful pain.

Dorothy

I'm forty-eight years old and a housewife. I had had some trouble with my jaw for about five years before I saw Dr. Gelb. I kept on being able to open it less and less. Then I started getting these pains down my neck and the sides of my throat. And my left arm bothered me. It was weak and sort of numb all of the time.

Of course, I didn't think that it had anything to do with my jaw. I thought it was a slipped disk or something. So I went to see a couple of specialists and they told me that it was nerves. They gave me some tranquilizers too. But I must have been allergic to them or something, because every time I took one, I started crying. Life didn't seem worth living. So I didn't take them anymore. Sometimes, though, when the pain got real bad, I would take a painkiller.

Like I said, I was having trouble with my jaw aside from all this pain. I didn't believe for a minute that it was in my head, like they told me. But what could I do? They were the experts. It made me very upset, though, and I was clenching my teeth a lot. Finally, my dentist sent me to Dr. Gelb to help my jaw.

Dr. Gelb stuck his fingers in my ears and I screamed. I thought I was going to die. And then he asked about all the other pain and said he could help. He put these broken tongue blades in my mouth to show me where the bite plate would position my teeth, and the pain started to go away. Just like that.

After I got the bite plate, the trouble in my jaw went away, I got back the strength and feeling in my left arm, and the pain didn't come back. Oh, I can open my mouth all the way again too.

Mary

I'm twenty-seven years old and work as an accountant. In 1974 I started having trouble with my eyes—blurry vision—and these terrible headaches. I went to an eye doctor three times until he practically threw me out, telling me that there was nothing physically wrong with my eyes.

After that I started seeing a million doctors. A sinus specialist, a neurologist, an internist. I kept on seeing new specialists and they all told me that there was nothing wrong with me.

Then I woke up one day with double vision. One of my eyes was paralyzed and I saw double. I was really scared at that point and went back to the eye doctor. He sent me to another doctor, a specialist, who told me that I had multiple sclerosis. One of the signs is one eye turning in. And my regular doctor accepted that verdict and tried to cheer me up. I was pretty recently married at the time, and it was a blow to my husband and me that we couldn't have a family. They tell you not to have children because you can pass the disease on, and because you could be an invalid all of a sudden. There is nothing they can do for you.

So for about eight months, I walked around with a patch over one of my eyes. That way I could see and get around. Then my cousin, a dentist, saw me and said that he thought I had this TMJ Syndrome, not multiple sclerosis. He said that you could see it because one side of my face was higher than the other. And he told me to go see Dr. Gelb.

Well, I hate being a victim. Anything was better than just sitting and waiting to become an invalid, so I went. Dr. Gelb said that my jaw was causing the problem and made a bite plate for me. And in four months, my eye straightened out, the double vision went away, the blurriness cleared up, and the headaches were relieved. I never had an incurable disease.

I have a good happy ending for this: I just found out today that I'm pregnant.

Etta

About four years ago, I started to have this problem with my ears. They would fill up and I'd have this terrible pressure and pain in them. The pain would go down my neck and along my jaw line. It was awful.

I went to a few doctors, mostly sinus specialists. Everyone thought that it was a sinus problem, but no one could find anything wrong with my ears. I had x-rays and all sorts of tests. No one could find anything. And no one could help the pain.

My daughter knew about my problem and I guess I had told her orthodontist something about it. Anyway, he suggested that I see Dr. Gelb. He knew him. I couldn't understand what my teeth had to do with the pain in my ears, but I was willing to try anything after the years of having this problem. Dr. Gelb explained how my jaw and body weren't balanced. My right leg was a little shorter than my left, and my bite was off on one side. Sure enough, a few days after he suggested placing a lift in the shoe to adjust for the short leg and adjusted my bite, the pain in my ears felt better.

Cheryl

I have had migraines since I was about three years old. They didn't come more than once or twice a month. By the time I came to Dr. Gelb's, I was having them two or three times a week. I knew that some were because of physical things, like my period. But others were due purely to emotional stress.

During all those years, you can imagine the myriad of tests I had and doctors that I saw. I've been hospitalized for blood tests, brain scans, electroencephalograms, every conceivable test to determine whether I had some disease or tumor. I didn't.

You learn to live with pain. It's the only way I knew. I had to take a lot of time off to fill myself with painkillers and wait for the endless headaches to subside enough for me to go on. But I got through school and then went to live in England for a while. I met and married a man there, and came back here. Sometimes the headaches would slow up in frequency. Sometimes they'd just come on and on again.

About six years ago, I was having a bad spell. It wasn't only hard on me, but on my husband too. We were having stupid fights because of all of the aggravation of me being sick all the time.

After one of these arguments, I left him in the dining room and locked myself in the bathroom. The headaches and arguments were just too much to handle. I was numb. I slit my wrists. Just like that.

In a little while, my husband came to see if something was wrong. He knocked on the door. I assumed that it wouldn't make any difference if I let him in. I was already dead. Of course, when he saw what I'd done, he called for an ambulance and wrapped my wrists in towels. I remember telling the doctor that he sewed very neatly.

Well, what was I supposed to do? It wasn't as if I wasn't trying to find help. No one, with their needles, pills and elaborate tests, could help me. So I got into the habit of calling my doctor whenever I got a bad headache, and being shot up with some drug that would knock me out until I felt better. Between shots, though, I was scared to go anywhere for fear that I'd get an attack in some crowded store or in a subway, where no one could help me.

Finally, last year, I heard about Dr. Gelb through a friend who had had pain in her neck and shoulders. Dr. Gelb had helped her out. I, too, had discomfort in those places aside from my headache. So I went to him.

I haven't had overnight relief. And I am glad about that. After you've suffered for as many years—twenty-six in all—as I have, you don't trust an overnight cure. But in the three and a half months that I've been under Dr. Gelb's care, I've had less frequent and less severe headaches. The pains in my shoulder and neck are gone. And I don't take the drugs that I used to take. It will take more time to make me completely well—not just physically, but emotionally as well. I'm just starting to go out again. I'm shopping all day today. For most people that would be a holiday, I guess. For me, it's a challenge.

Ena

A few years back, I was hit on the ear, I had an accident. For a day and a half, I couldn't hear anything out of that ear and it was terribly painful. But the pain cleared up, so I didn't pay any attention to it. This was in the early seventies. And for the next few years, whenever I was dunked under water, you know, if I was swimming, I would get a pain in that ear. But that was all.

Then one day I took a shower and washed my hair, and water got into that ear. The pain was tremendous. It was like a knife going into my body. The only doctor I had then was a gynecologist, and she gave me some painkillers and sent me to the hospital. When they examined my ear, they found that I had a punctured eardrum and needed an operation.

I had the operations, four in all, and the pain never stopped from that point on. I went to specialist after specialist and each one told me that the ear had healed fine. They said that my hearing was perfect too. Well, my ear gave me tremendous pain and I couldn't hear out of it—regardless of what they said.

I went back to the doctor who operated on me and he said, "I know what's wrong with you, and it's not in your ears. Have you had bad pains in your legs?" I told him I had, and he said that I had rheumatism. So I took medicine for that. Then one side of my face started to hurt and they said that it was neuralgia and gave me pills for that. And then I started having pains in my heart. But nobody could make the pains go away. So I relied on the painkillers.

I didn't have much choice. I'm a mother and a working woman. I have two children depending on me and, at that time, a job in which I dealt with people all day. Finally, I found a specialist who wasn't willing to give up until he found the reason for my pain. Thank God for him. He sent me to a number of specialists, all of whom said that after the operations I had had, I should expect a certain amount of pain. My doctor didn't think that was so and he eventually sent me to Dr. Gelb.

I had heard so many stories about what was causing the pain, and this one about the jaw didn't sound any more believable than the rest. But then, Dr. Gelb put the appliance in my mouth and I could feel something pulling. Not an unpleasant sensation. Just a pulling on the muscles around my jaw and ear. After the second or third visit, the pain in my ear starting gradually easing, a little more every day. In a month I forgot that I ever had a pain. It was completely gone. And the pain in my chest and legs was better too.

Obdulia

I'm fifty-five. I had a good job in the maintenance department of a large office building until all my problems started. I remember just how they started too. In the fall of 1976, I was given a new floor and was told to vacuum the rooms too. Vacuuming is a man's job. That machine is too heavy for me. But I did it anyway. After a few weeks, though, I'd work for an hour and start to get dizzy. Then I'd just pass out. I was so white that some of the other ladies thought I was dead. And this happened every night after that. I would work for an hour or so and pass out.

My doctor told me to rest for a few days and I did. But the same thing happened when I went back to work. Then the pain started. The whole side of my head ached so bad, all I could do was sit and hold it. I couldn't bend or walk or even bathe myself anymore. I just sat in bed for two months.

Then I tried to go back to work, but the same pain and fainting spells happened. The doctors thought maybe it was sinus because I had to breathe through my mouth and my nose was always running. They did tests, but didn't find anything.

One day when I was going to the hospital for tests, I fell down because of the dizziness. One of the doctors who knew me saw me and was afraid I had a tumor. He said that I couldn't go back to work at all. I spent a week in the hospital for the tests and then five months at home in bed. Everything I ate, I threw up. I was an invalid.

Finally, one of my doctors suggested I see Dr. Gelb. I was practically carried into the office. He pinched and poked around while I screamed from the pain. Then he put a splint in my mouth and injected all the trigger points in the muscles in my neck and jaw. I started feeling better.

I haven't been back to work yet, but the pain in my head is gone and so is the pain in my shoulder and back. I can eat again and have gained back forty pounds. I still can't go out by myself, but I can bathe and dress and am not in such horrible pain. When I just think about that awful pain, I start to cry.

Carol

I'm thirty-five and have been having problems on and off with my jaw since I was twenty-two. I was in college at that time and went to kiss someone, when my jaw went out. From that point on, it clicked when I opened or closed it.

I knew something was wrong because I couldn't open my mouth very wide without feeling a lot of pain, but I never did anything about it for some time. It didn't bother me that much on a day-to-day level, and I don't like going to doctors frequently. But as the years went by, I started to have an increasing amount of pain in the right side of my face, spreading up to the top of my head and going down the back of my neck. And my mouth opened less and less widely.

One day I was supposed to have this staff meeting with our vice-president and I realized that the pain was really making it difficult to even talk. I managed to get through the meeting and even open my mouth wide enough to drink some coffee, but I couldn't get it around a sandwich.

That was Thanksgiving weekend and I had to wait to see my dentist until the following Monday. So I saw another dentist. He told me that I had an extreme spasm in my right jaw that was so bad that he couldn't even get near me to do definitive tests. Eventually he got the x-rays that he needed and found that I'd thrown my jaw way out of place, probably in my sleep or when I yawned. It had been out of place for some time, and he suggested that I wear a permanent plate in my mouth.

I refused to wear the plate, but said that I would do some exercises and wear a night guard, which I did. And I was careful not to sleep on the right side, which always triggered off another attack. I began to find, however, that many other things triggered off that terrible pain, such as air conditioners and drafts on that side of my face. Even a peck on that cheek. If I slept on the right side, I'd wake up in pain. If I slept on the left side, a draft would cause the pain to start and I'd wake up that way too. I couldn't find a comfortable place to rest.

I have a very high-pressure job, and the pain was making it more difficult for me to be effective, and more tense about being effective. I was taking painkillers and anti-inflammatory medicines. But the pain was always there. Finally, I got fed up and went to see Dr. Gelb.

He told me the same things that my first dentist told me, that I had to have a splint to reposition my jaw, but this time I agreed to wear it. At this point, I was much more irritable than I used to be. Pain makes you supersensitive after a while. I was also sensitive to light and sound. Even the sound at a movie seemed uncomfortably loud. And my eyes and ears had started to become affected. My balance was off. I was falling down a lot—something that I just don't do normally.

I would say that it took about a month for the pain level to go down after the splint was put in my mouth. A couple of changes occurred right away. For instance, I was able to sleep on my right side just a few days after the bite plate went in. Then, slowly, the dull, ever-present pain in my neck and head and shoulders and back began to dissipate. I still have some discomfort in my neck and back, which Dr. Gelb says is common until the muscles are comfortable in their new position. I just can't wait for the whole treatment to be over. I just can't wait until I don't ever have to think about my jaw or feel this pain again.

Patty

About three years ago, my jaw started cracking. It was very noticeable, and at times it was painful. Then my jaw started getting stuck when I was eating. It would freeze and I would have to force it open. Then the pain got really bad. It was in the back of my jaw, and I was getting headaches—especially when my jaw would get stuck.

I went to a number of doctors. First, my regular doctor said that there was nothing really wrong and that my jaw would just start feeling better. Then I went to two dentists and they told me the same thing. Finally, I saw an oral surgeon, who sent me to another dentist, and he put a mouthpiece in my mouth. The plate was way too high, and seemed to make the whole problem even worse. Finally, he said that I should see Dr. Gelb. By this time, my back and shoulders were also sore and ached a lot.

Dr. Gelb said that the last dentist had tried to balance my teeth, instead of balancing the jaws. He found that not only my jaws were unbalanced, but my legs were too. I put a lift in one shoe and began to wear the appliance that Dr. Gelb made. Of course, he treated the muscles in my neck and shoulder, which were all in spasm from walking around unbalanced like that for so long.

My jaw is much better now. I don't have the clicking anymore. Most of the pain in my neck, shoulders and head is gone, but when I eat a hard roll, or pick up something heavy, I can knock the balance out and have another headache. The most important part of the treatment for me is that the pain is gone away. I don't get so impatient or snappy now.

Irene

I'm thirty-nine. I've had this problem since I was about twenty. I've been shuttled from doctor to dentist to neurologist to psychiatrist to just about any medical professional. Name the field; I've been referred there for treatment.

I had a pain in my jaw. It was like a toothache where I had no tooth. It throbbed and throbbed. That's when I started on my circuit of doctors. I lost a lot of teeth going to dentists. The pain seemed to come from a tooth, and because they didn't know what else to do, they yanked it—and the one next to it, and the one next to that one, and on and on.

I had been in the hospital for three weeks for tests. They were trying to see if it was some kind of neuralgia. Then they did this freezing procedure. They go through a sinus opening in your cheek and inject the nerve. They do this while you're awake. You get an analgesic before they inject you, and then they strap you to a table. But the analgesic didn't work for me. I passed out. They hit too many nerves and froze one whole side of my face. Then they sent me home. That was it. They sent me home, twenty pounds lighter. So I figured that I was off doctors for a while.

The pain continued on and off for ten years. I managed to live with it. Then, when I was thirty, I opened my mouth the wrong way one night, and the next day I couldn't open it at all. From that point on, everything went really wild. That's when the pain went into the jaw joint. I went to my dentist in a panic. He referred me to someone who said that he could help me for ten thousand dollars. Who has that kind of money?

I was on baby food for three months, and I had a cotton ball in between my teeth so that I wouldn't use that joint. Being a legal secretary and on the phone a lot, this wasn't too helpful. I went to rheumatologists, psychiatrists and orthopedic men. Many of them told me to get married and all my problems would go away. One orthopedic specialist said that he didn't like to do it, but he could remove the bad joint and then take out the good one so that I'd be even. I said, "Forget it." At this point, you have very little faith left. I still had the pain and couldn't get my mouth open fully. And I was beginning to doubt my mind as well.

In my mid thirties, I was able to eat a little and talk when necessary. I was living on painkillers and tranquilizers. I went to another pain clinic and was treated by one of the first neurologists I'd gone to about fifteen years before. He said, "Well, you've made it this far." As if, you know, how dare I expect to be treated when it was obvious that I could survive with the pain.

Finally, one of my dentist's colleagues suggested that I come to Dr. Gelb. When I walked into his office, he examined me and told me what was wrong and where the pain was. He knew exactly what was wrong with me. It was a real shock to have someone say, "You're a classic case. We deal with this all of the time."

After four or five months of wearing the splint and having my muscles treated, I felt a big difference. The throbbing in my jaw went away. I could open my mouth. I still don't eat very chewy things like apples. Hopefully, I will be able to, although I'm a little frightened of trying. I've hurt myself before.

I'm about 60 to 70 percent better. I hope to get even better, though I'm quite satisfied with that. The alternative—and this is what really drove me here—was that they wanted to sever the nerve. And then I would have had total numbness. I don't think that I would like to live like that.

John

I'm twenty-four years old and am a student at Yale University. Right now I'm on a medical leave of absence, with only one year left to go.

I had to leave school because of a severe pain around the temples. My head, my temples and my whole face were tremendously swollen. The pain was so bad that I just couldn't sleep. I couldn't function on any level at all. It's hard to say when the problem started. I have allergies and have had a couple of sinus infections. The doctors have always attributed all my problems to sinuses. So I had an operation for that. They drilled a hole through the bone near my sinus to make sure that the sinus wouldn't get clogged and infected. I had that operation two summers before I came to see Dr. Gelb. When I got out of the hospital, though, I still had a lot of pain. The surgeon and sinus specialists at home didn't know what to think, so they sent me to a neurologist. He just mumbled and grumbled about tension and gave me something for my emotional problems. What emotional problems? I didn't have any until I started gaining the forty pounds from the drug he gave me.

Obviously, the drug didn't help me, but it made me sleepy all the time. The pain was so bad that I just had to leave school, which I did. I went back to my dentist at home and he said that he knew how to treat me. "Oh, I can do that very easily." And he gave me an appliance to wear. I wore it for two and a half months, but it wasn't helping. So I went back to him and told him so. He just didn't understand the problem that well, I guess. I was only the second patient that he'd tried to help. Anyway, he told me that I had really severe emotional problems and that was causing the pain. Was that also causing the whole side of my face to swell up?

The dentist also said that he didn't know what good it would do, but he'd refer me to Dr. Gelb. He just wanted to get me off his back.

He treated me in the usual manner, with a splint and muscle therapy. And it worked. Gradually the pain in my temples went away and so did the swelling. I stopped taking the drugs I was on and lost the forty pounds a lot slower than they went on. Oh, sure, I still have some discomfort. But now I can take an aspirin and go on. I think that in two or three months, I'll be pain-free. But I'm happy with the way I am for now. I expect to be back in school again for the next semester.

Debbie

I'm twenty-six and I work in a publishing company. This is the first time in years that I've been able to hold down a full-time job.

When I got out of college, I started to have what seemed like spasms in my mouth. They throbbed so strongly, like a heartbeat in my mouth. The pain was near my wisdom teeth, and the area around there was swollen, but I had already had them out, so it couldn't have been that. I saw my orthodontist and oral surgeon, and both said that nothing was wrong with my teeth. Finally, my dentist thought that I was grinding my teeth at night and that was causing the pain. He gave me a plastic bite plate to wear at night to stop the grinding. It didn't help and it made me nauseous, so I stopped wearing it.

My family and everyone else were saying that it was all because of tension, that it was all psychological. Some days the pain would be bad, and some days it would be minor, but it never went away. Finally, a friend of the family suggested that I go to this TMJ clinic to see if that was the problem. But they didn't treat me like Dr. Gelb did.

I went to this clinic and they asked me all these psychological questions. Was I nervous? Did I love my mother? Was it hard living at home? Well, I had been through a pretty bad time in the months preceding the visit, but I'd been through bad times before. It was the pain that was driving me nuts.

They took an impression of my teeth and poked around a little. I definitely had a muscle spasm in my jaw. They gave me a series of jaw exercises and some tranquilizers. I did those exercises every night and took the drug, but they didn't help. Finally, after three weeks, I came in the clinic in such pain and said, "Please, you've got to help me. You've got to treat me." The head of the clinic said, "O.K.," and sprayed my mouth with some numbing stuff. Then he waved goodbye.

After that, I went back to refill the prescription for the tranquilizers. I just got as many refills as I wanted. In the meantime, my neck and shoulders were so tight that it felt like the muscles were ropes being twisted tight. I was getting worse. The pain was terrible. Nothing was stopping it. So finally, I thought that they were right. Maybe it was psychological. And I went to see a psychologist. That didn't help.

Just when I was giving up hope, a friend of mine who had had trouble with her jaw suggested that I visit Dr. Gelb. I was hesitant, but I was so fed up with the pain that I decided to go. Dr. Gelb took x-rays of my jaw and told me exactly what was wrong and how he would treat it. He made a plate for me, and within two to three months I was 90 percent better. The pain and swelling in my mouth were gone, and so were the spasms in my neck and shoulders.

Robert

I'm an attorney. I started getting these severe headaches and pains in my face about a year ago. The pains came in waves across the front of my face near the temples, and sometimes in my ears. At one point, I took a plane to certain meetings two and three times a week. The pain in my ears was so bad and lasted so long that I had to stop flying to these conferences. Not very good for business.

I started to see some doctors about the problem. A few thought that it was migraines. My doctor said that I was working too hard and prescribed tranquilizers. He told me to take it easy. Then he sent me to get checked by an ear, nose and throat specialist, who found an infection in my sinuses. That cleared up fine, but the pain remained.

So my doctor sent me to another ear, nose and throat specialist. This one found a chronic inflammation in my throat. They did a biopsy and started to treat that. But the headaches never were relieved.

In the midst of all of this, I saw a neurologist, who did a whole series of tests to check for some organic dysfunction in the brain. Everything was normal. But the neurologist also said that I was working too hard, that perhaps I wasn't meant to be an attorney. Maybe I should terminate my practice and become a librarian in a small town in Maine. Maybe I should see a psychologist.

So I saw a psychologist. He, unlike all these other specialists, thought that I handled my life style very well. But my original doctor was sure that I was manic depressive. So I got a new doctor. He was not at all convinced that my throat or my sinuses were affecting my headaches. And he sent me to Dr. Gelb.

Dr. Gelb just looked at me and said, "I know what your problem is." He could see from the misalignment of my features that my jaw was off. Of course, I was skeptical. Everyone, after all, thought they knew what my problem was. Dr. Gelb put gauze between my teeth and told me to bite down. He said that in five minutes I would start to feel relief.

Sure.

In a couple of minutes, the sharp pain started to disappear. Then the soreness dissipated too. Since that first visit, I haven't had a severe headache.

After I started wearing the plate, my neck started bothering me. Dr. Gelb said that the discomfort was normal and it would go away. It did. And my ears cleared up too.

I'm not doubting my ability to practice or my sanity any longer. For a while, I was thinking of selling my house and moving to a slower kind of community than New York City. I don't need to. Just like the psychologist said, I'm handling my hectic life style pretty well.

Michaelina

I was run over by a car three years ago. I was crossing the street, was hit and thrown forty feet in the air. Then I was thrown back against a car going the opposite way. Everyone thought that I wouldn't pull through. But after nine months in the hospital wearing a brace from my neck to the bottom of my legs, I was able to come home. The doctors said that my body had healed, but I was in constant pain.

I had had a severe concussion, and no matter what painkillers they gave me in the hospital, the pain was constantly there. I couldn't sleep, and I was clenching my teeth. When I got home, I still had constant headaches and terrible pains in my jaw. Nobody could touch my shoulders or my back, they were both so sore. And no doctor could tell me what was wrong. I went to twenty-one of the finest specialists in the country, and no one could help me. They suggested I go to a psychiatrist and learn to live with it.

I'm an actress. It's torture for me to sit at home. So I was trying to get back in the swing of things right after I got home. I learned to walk with canes and crutches, and finally was able to support myself, to the amazement of many of the doctors who treated me. But the pain was still crippling me. I was seeing chiropractors, acupuncturists, taking pills. You name it. Nothing helped. I also noticed that something peculiar had happened to my face. I had new pictures taken and saw that my face had aged terribly, and that my jaw had receded. Had I grown that old and disfigured from the accident?

I have a friend, an announcer, who had been seeing Dr. Gelb for treatment of a jaw problem, and he thought that maybe Dr. Gelb could help me. I was skeptical. After all, I'd seen the best, the most well-known specialists in the country; why would a dentist be able to help me? But I went along to the appointment anyway, to see how a treatment worked on my friend.

While he was having some spasms broken up in his shoulders, I was sitting on a stool, clenching my teeth against the pain as usual. Dr. Gelb turned to me and said, ''You're in pain, aren't you?'' I said, ''Yes.'' And then he examined me a little. Oh, God, every place he touched on my shoulders and my back made me scream. Finally, I said, ''I don't need you to give me any more problems. I've had enough pain in the last two years.'' He said that if I'd just trust him, he'd help me.

I let him inject and break up the spasms in my neck, shoulders and back. As I was leaving, I suddenly had this incredible feeling. I can't really explain it. I was free of pain for the first time since the accident. I went home and slept for twenty-four hours, just like that, with my clothes on and everything.

When I woke up, I called Dr. Gelb and made an appointment to have the whole treatment. He gave me a bite plate that restored my chin's original position and wiped off the lines of age that I'd suddenly accumulated after the accident. My muscles were treated, and the pain was relieved permanently. I would see Dr. Gelb once every few months just for a checkup.

Then I got this earache. It was horrible. I thought that it was connected to some kind of sinus infection, and I went to an ear, nose and throat specialist. He said there was nothing wrong with my ears or sinuses, but did I have any dental troubles? I said, "Funny you should ask. I have been seeing Dr. Gelb for my jaw." And he said that he was just going to suggest that I see Dr. Gelb. So I made an appointment and had my bite plate built up where I had worn it down, and sure enough, the pain went away.

Alicia

I'm twenty-seven now, and work as a registered nurse. Just a year ago, I was working and living in Houston, Texas. One day, when I was having lunch in the cafeteria with my friends, I suddenly lost my hearing. It was as though the air conditioning unit went berserk and got really loud. There was a roaring in my ears. I kept commenting on it to my friends, but they didn't hear it as loud as I did. I was really having trouble hearing people speak. We got up from lunch and went outside, but the noise in my ears didn't go away.

I went back to the office and told the doctor I was working for about it. He checked my ears and found nothing wrong. Then he called an associate and made an appointment for me to have a hearing test. Between that lunch incident and the test, I had grown used to the ringing and roaring, I guess. So when the doctor came out and told me that I was 90 percent deaf in my right ear, I was stunned. He wanted to go ahead and put me in the hospital, thinking that maybe I was stricken by some disease that causes sudden deafness.

I was on the pill at that time, and it seems that bloodclotting has something to do with the deafness, so the doctors felt even more that this was the case, and put me in the hospital for five days. They did all kinds of tests, which turned out negative. Then they tried this blocking procedure which I never heard of. They injected Xylocaine into my neck to hit all the nerve endings, to numb them. Hopefully, that would open the ear. It was the most pain that I'd experienced in my life, and the procedure was repeated for three consecutive days. It didn't do a thing for my hearing.

I was sent home, taken off the pill, and told that I just had to live with the problem. So I did. The hearing problem really disturbed me. It was like everyone talked in a tunnel. I wasn't used to it. On one side I heard perfectly. My other side didn't exist.

One day, the office was very busy. I was on the phone all morning, then I went to lunch. I was sitting there, and then I passed out. I never really lost consciousness; I just kind of fell over. I felt like I'd been drinking and woke up not knowing where I was.

My doctor took my blood pressure and checked the other vital signs. They were all normal. He sent me to a neurologist in the emergency room at the hospital. The neurologist checked me out from head to toe and said that he was going to admit me because there was a possibility that I had a brain tumor.

In the hospital, I had brain scans, spinal taps, all kinds of complicated tests. I was starting to get headaches and dizziness more frequently. But all the reports were negative.

I went to New Jersey to visit my mother for six weeks. At this point the headaches were really severe and I spent the whole time in bed. And the pain was starting to travel down my neck and back. So I called the neurologist in Houston and he said that I'd better get back there for more tests. Those tests came out normal, so I was sent to an internist to be checked out. He found a low-grade fever and a slight swelling of the glands in my neck, which had no noticeable cause, and put me back in the hospital for another battery of tests.

They operated on my neck and took out some of the lymph nodes to test for certain rare and lethal diseases. All those tests and the blood tests that they did were, again, normal. And then they told me that the problem was probably psychological.

I was getting a divorce right after I'd given birth to twin girls. I had been separated for almost a year, and the divorce was being finalized in two months. So the doctors said that I was under too much stress. But I wasn't. I was very happy with my decision, and led a well-organized, satisfying life. The doctors wouldn't believe that. They wanted me to take tranquilizers four times a day. But I didn't need them, so I didn't take them.

Then one day, while I was waiting to see the internist, I noticed an article about the TMJ Syndrome in a magazine. I brought it in to the doctor and asked him if he thought that my problem could be caused by this. He just brushed it off as a new fad.

No one could help me, and I was in too much pain to work or take care of my kids, so I went back home to New Jersey. All this took place in about eight months, from April through December. It was getting near the holidays, I remember, and I went to see my dentist. Just to have some cavities filled. Again, in his waiting room, I saw an article about the TMJ Syndrome and it sounded exactly like what I had. The article said that your dentist could tell you if you had it, so I asked mine. He thought that I did and said that I'd probably have to see this specialist he knew in New York, but first he wanted to try some treatment methods.

This dentist ground down my teeth—the exact opposite of what I needed. After almost two months of this, I had one of my bad headaches and called the dentist up, demanding the name of a specialist. Finally, I went to see Dr. Gelb.

I had the x-rays taken and the standard examination. Dr. Gelb said that he believed he knew what was wrong. But a lot of people had told me that they knew what was wrong when they didn't. And many of their diagnoses were more acceptable to me than this one. After all, for the range of symptoms I had, and the severity of them, you'd expect to need an operation, to have something major taken out or put in. All Dr. Gelb wanted to do was put a plate in my mouth.

Finally, out of desperation, I agreed to the treatment. My hopes were not up at all. And the first few weeks that I had the plate in, it hurt me so badly that I was sure it was doing more damage than good. Now I wouldn't dare take it out of my mouth. My headaches are gone and so is the pain in my neck and shoulders. Fifty percent of my hearing has been restored in that one ear, though I still have bouts of dizziness and ringing in the ears, especially if my plate needs adjusting.

I'm one of the lucky ones, though. I got here. I'm in the medical profession and none of the concerned doctors I work with could help me. I'm not putting them down, but in order to get help, I practically had to go outside the conventional medical system. All of my experience only helped me maintain my resolve that the problem wasn't a mental one. Just think of the people without a medical education.

I'm back at work now. One of the first things I did when I was getting better was to send reprints of articles about the TMJ Syndrome to my doctors in Houston. Maybe my experience can save other patients from going through the same thing.

Susan

Thirteen years ago, I had a kidney operation, and that's when this long horror story began. At the time, I was forty, happily married and holding down a good job.

One doctor said that I needed to have the kidney out, but another doctor, a new one, wanted to try and save the kidney. He experimented with various treatments, for which I was in the hospital every three or four weeks. Then he said that he thought he'd treated me successfully, only I'd have to go in the hospital every so often to get checked.

Then I was getting worse and worse. I went back to the doctor and he said he wanted to try a new medicine on me. It would make me lose my teeth, but I agreed. I was very sick and wanted help. I did lose my top teeth at a very young age, and got dentures. That was three or four years after the kidney operation failed.

Right after that, I started having this awful pain in my jaws. It was so bad that I couldn't do my work well. Then I started fighting with my husband. I had this pain in my mouth and I didn't know what was wrong. He thought it was all in my head.

Somehow I kept working. Ten hours a day. My husband and I kept fighting. Then one day, we got in an accident, my son, my daughter, my husband and I. I was the only one that was hurt. My back was hurt, and I ended up in a hospital for three months.

Eventually the pain in my jaw, and the pain in my back, and my husband and I battling all of the time caused me to lose my job. Everybody started saying that I should see a psychiatrist. They thought that the trouble started because I was arguing with my husband. But the pain was there before.

Anyway, I went to this psychiatrist and he finally decided to give me shock treatments for the pain in my face. I had ninety-eight shock treatments. Well, I just couldn't take it anymore, so one day I decided to leave home. I couldn't take the strain of arguing and the pain. My husband called up the doctor and said that the psychiatrist wanted to talk to me. I agreed to see him, like a fool.

I went to this doctor in a combination nursing home and rest home. We were waiting in the lobby, and all of a sudden, the doctor comes over to me with a nurse and says, "Come on." "Where are you taking me?" I asked him. And he said, "Come on. Don't give me any trouble." So I went with him, tears streaming down my face from the pain I was in. He put me in this room all by myself and I was pleading with him, "Doctor, I'm in so much pain." And he said that I was not. I started fighting him. You know, I wanted to get out of there. Then he put a strait jacket on me and left me there all night long alone, crying and screaming. No calls. I couldn't even call my mother and tell her where I was. They kept me there for two weeks.

Finally, I said to one of the nurses that if the doctor didn't come to see me immediately, I'd make her sorry that they ever saw me there. They let me go in to see him and I said, "Doctor, am I mentally ill?" And he said, "No." And I asked him if I was physically ill, and he said that he didn't know. I told him that nerves don't make you have a fever. They don't make your face swell up. I said that he was keeping me there against my will and I could sue him for that. He said that he knew and that was why he was letting me go.

I could have sued him but good, but I was too sick. I was even too sick to leave my home. I couldn't work to support myself. So I went home. My husband still didn't believe that I was sick. Then one night, I was holding my head in my hands, begging him to find someone to help me, and he said, "O.K. Tomorrow morning we'll take you in for more shock treatments." I didn't know what else to do, so I went.

One night the pain got so bad that I really thought I would kill myself. I was admitted into a hospital for two weeks, and my doctor there sent me to a specialist. An ear, nose and throat specialist. This new doctor examined me and saw that I was in terrible pain. He gave me a needle in my jaw that numbed the pain. For two weeks, I felt so good. But then the medicine wore off, and I went back to the doctor. When he saw that the pain was still there, he put me in the hospital.

The next morning, he came in and said, "Susan, we are going to take you downstairs and going to give you a test. Your husband and sister-in-law will be present." Not knowing what the test was, I agreed. He wheeled me downstairs and took this long wire or tube. He started shoving it down my nose. He just kept shoving and shoving. I was screaming so loud, I must have awakened half the building. I scared my husband and his sister so that they ran out of the building. And when he finished pushing this thing down one side, he said that he had to do the other.

Finally, when he finished, he said, "Don't worry, Susan. I'm going to fix you up right now. I'm going to give you a needle and the pain is going to go away." I was in so much pain, I thought I was going to die. He shot me on both sides of my face, in my mouth and outside. He put me in a wheelchair and we were going up the elevator. I kept looking at him, waiting for the pain to go away. But it never went away. "How long does this medicine take to work?" I asked. He said that I'd feel fine in a moment. But I didn't. And I started thinking that I must be crazy. Why wasn't the needle working?

We got to my room and he said, "How do you feel?" Tears were running down my face. "How do you feel, Susan?" I said that I wasn't going to tell because he wouldn't believe me. He said "Try me." I said, "Doctor, I still have the pain." And he told me that was fine, because he didn't give me anything but water. He wanted to find out if I really had pain or if I was crazy.

Then he came in the next day and said they were going to operate on my sinuses. Scrape away some scar tissue and put plastic windows in there. I thought that that tube going down my nose was the worst pain I'd ever feel, but after the operation, the pain was worse.

After three months, I was just as bad as when I got out of the hospital. They sent me to a specialist because they didn't know what was wrong with me. He put me on three different kinds of tranquilizers which seemed to make the pain more bearable.

The next thing that happened is that my husband lost his job and I, with all my pain, had to go back to work. The doctor said that I was too sick, but my family insisted.

I was still in so much pain and so sick. To get through the days, I just kept on taking more and more tranquilizers. Finally, I lost that job when they rushed me to the hospital. When they saw what kind of drugs I was taking, they said that it was lucky I was alive. The medications were slowly killing my brain. I was becoming a robot. They cleared my system of the drugs, but they couldn't do anything for the pain. My husband was telling me that I was crazy. I was so sick that I just wanted to go on the medication again.

Then one day, I was driving and my husband saw me stopped at a light. He was with a friend, who couldn't believe how bad I looked. Then this friend suggested I go see a specialist on Staten Island. I was home that day and really sick. My husband came home and found me lying on the living room floor. He saw me there and said, "Well, what the hell is the matter with you?" I couldn't even talk, I was in so much pain. He said, "Well, I'm not losing my job for you," and turns around and walks out the door. My mind was all fuzzy and I thought: What am I going to do? I crawled into the kitchen and knocked the phone off the hook and dialed my sister. I just said her name and passed out, but she knew it was trouble and called the police. What I'd had was a heart seizure. I could have died.

After that, my husband took me to this new doctor and he sent me to Dr. Gelb. Dr. Gelb examined me once and said that the denture made for my upper teeth was not right, and that was causing all the trouble. He injected my muscles and fixed my teeth. I didn't get better immediately. But that's O.K. If it happened too fast, I'd be afraid that the pain would come back. I don't have it every day, though. Some days I don't have it at all.

You don't know what that means after thirteen years. I feel like a new girl, like a new person. I feel like singing and going out dancing in the street.

14

Postscript

This book reflects my belief that the majority of headaches, backaches and other chronic muscular pain are not psychosomatic, but are somatopsychic instead.

Psychosomatic disturbances are real. People with deep emotional disturbances can experience all kinds of physical ills. However, the application of this diagnosis to everything for which a physician can find no pathological origin has caused thousands of people to suffer needlessly for years. Not only do they suffer physically, but they suffer emotionally as well, since they are always doubting the veracity of their discomfort. They feel guilty for burdening family and friends with their continual, painful trauma.

I have found that most chronic pain has a physical foundation. It may not be a disease that will show up on a lab test or an x-ray, but a hand pressed on the painful area often reveals a spasm or trigger point. Can the millions of patients who sit in waiting rooms throughout this country all have mental disorders so gross that they result in muscles twisted into spasms or joints forced out of balance? We don't think so.

The approach, as demonstrated in this book, proves again and again that we are all born with or soon develop small physical imperfections, some of which mature and cause a weak link in the skeletal system. Sometimes this weak link can be aggravated by an accident or some other injury. That area, be it in the shoulders, the jaw or the back, will not be able to withstand even the normal stresses of daily life—dietary, environmental, as well as emotional.

A weak link may not cause pain for years, but it still stresses the rest of the system continually. When a spasm finally does occur, you can't blame it on some emotional upheaval alone. There's obviously a physical factor.

I'm not saying that emotions are not a great part of these chronic pain problems. However, for most of our patients, the physical predisposition to the chronic disorder was present long before the pain started. The stress of work, school, love, whatever, may never have elicited any discomfort if the predisposing physical weakness hadn't been there in the body. That's why I feel that somatopsychic is a far more correct label for most chronic pain disorders.

Aside from giving reassurance that most chronic muscular pain is not due to mental illness, I wanted to stir the reader to evaluate the health care that he or she is getting. Our medical system is the best in the world, but it can work only if the patient is an active partner in treatment. Ask questions. Get more than one evaluation. And most of all, if one physician can't help you, don't feel that you've failed. Look for help elsewhere. Read up on your symptoms so that you know where to go for help. As with everything else, the more you put into your health care, the more you'll get out of it.

Index

243